The Nutrient-Dense Diet

The Metabolic Key to Unlocking Weight Loss

By
D. Lewis

Author and Publisher
D. Lewis
docdawa@gmail.com

Graphics and Book Layout
Peter Brooks Hale

ISBN-13:
978-1508528555
ISBN-10:
1508528551

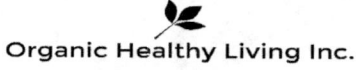

Organic Healthy Living Inc.
Publications
2015

The Nutrient-Dense Diet

The Metabolic Key to Unlocking Weight Loss

You are what you eat....

The Nutrient-Dense Solution
For Unlocking Cellular Dormancy

The Nutrient-Dense Diet
The Metabolic Key to Unlocking Weight Loss

Table of Contents

Forward

Losing weight- and keeping it off- is one of the most frustrating and challenging ordeals that many of us face. Yet it doesn't have to be that difficult. All around us we see slender, energetic people who are no different than us. You too can have the body you want- all you need is to relearn a few basic principles of nutrition.

The Nutrient-Dense Diet is different from most of the weight loss programs and plans out there today. The NDD is not a "quick fix" solution based on gimmicks or fad diets. It doesn't even require you to count calories or grams of anything. Instead it is a modern blend of solid science and common sense based on the basic principle that quality foods can help get your metabolism "back on track."

You CAN lose weight. And you deserve it! No one is doomed to be unhealthy or severely overweight. It is not in our genes to be obese. Too many of us are simply eating inappropriately for our biochemistry- and as a result our metabolisms are powered down- a condition I call "cellular dormancy". "Unlocking" cellular dormancy is the key to lasting weight loss and is easily done. This book will give you the information and tools you need to re-boot your metabolism. Think of it as your very own "metabolic makeover" guide and personal coach.

The Nutrient-Dense Diet is much more than just a "diet". Instead, it is a complete lifestyle and eating plan designed to support and empower you to "take back your life" from the corporate food giants who control and market the vast majority of our food choices today. It will teach you why this is so important and show you exactly how to do it.

Nutrient-Dense foods are far less processed, much less adulterated, and significantly more nutritious than their SAD (Standard American Diet) counterparts. Changing your diet *will*

1

change your metabolism- so you can burn calories and turn them into the energy you need, rather than storing them as fat.

When it comes to your body and your health, you deserve the best. Health is something everyone values and wants. When we are healthy and fit most of life's challenges are much more manageable. But if our health is lost, we can have money, relationships, prestige, possessions, etc. but they will be much harder to enjoy. Good health contributes hugely to a happier state of mind. The Nutrient-Dense Diet strives to help you achieve a healthy body in which to house a creative, happy, loving mind. Isn't this what we all want? Well guess what? It's within your reach!

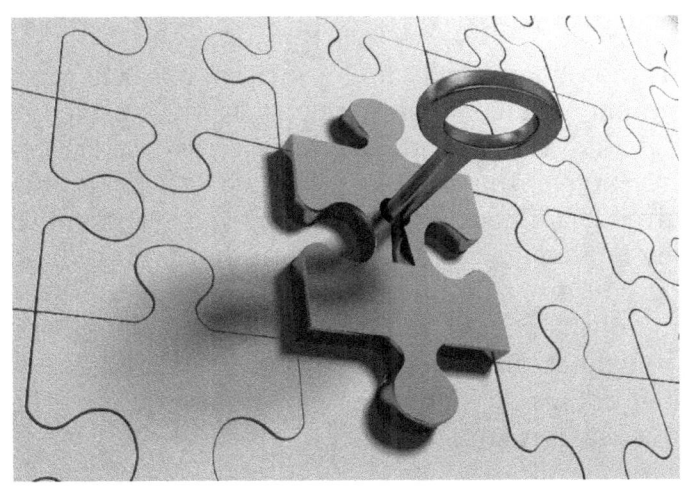

Introduction

Unlocking The Weight Dilemma

You are about to read a completely new approach to the dilemma of weight gain. This book holds the key to unlocking the main reason why so many people today are struggling as never before with weight issues. And the solution may surprise you!

Most "diet" books and programs today are capable of getting results- for a while. Unfortunately- as we all know- most of us end up in the "yo-yo" effect. Our weight goes down, but it all too quickly comes back up again. This book can show you how to stop yo-yoing once and for all!

Most diets and weight loss programs only work while you are on them. Stop the "quick fix" method, and the weight comes back, often really quickly. Why? The disconcerting reason is simple: quick fixes don't work for more than the short term. And the reason is as obvious as it is simple: they don't address the underlying problem or issue.

So what is the underlying issue for most of us? I am going to give you a two-part answer. The first part of the answer is..... *your metabolism*. And the second part, for the vast majority of people is....*the type of food you eat.* And guess what? The second answer, "food", directly influences the first answer, "metabolism". And this is why most quick fix diet solutions don't work for very long- because if you don't permanently change your diet to optimize your metabolism, then if you go back to your old way of eating, nothing substantial has changed. This is where "The Nutrient-Dense Diet" comes in. If your food is "smart" then it will be your friend –the way it is supposed to be!

This book will give you all the information you need to know to take charge of your diet, your life, and your metabolism- not for the short term, but for the rest of your life. The concepts I will present here make sense, are scientifically accurate, are tried and true, and are surprisingly simple. If you are really, truly serious about "taking back your life" and getting a grip on your metabolism from "the inside out" this program will change your life! I hesitate to say this, because so many of us have heard this sort of claim before. The difference is, this program is a potent combination of good science and common sense- not hype. And common sense, coupled with a good sound basic understanding of how our bodies burn calories and create energy (metabolism 101) is a powerful combination that can get amazing results!

Now a word of warning (uh oh!). As I said in the beginning, this is not a "QUICK FIX" plan. That does NOT mean it works slowly- on the contrary, most people get amazingly quick results. When I say it is not a quick fix, I really mean that it is more of a long term, lifestyle fix. If you are ready to actually change some of your approaches to food, and are interested in learning how to have a healthier eating lifestyle, then this book is for you. However, if you are totally happy with how and what you eat, and have no desire or interest in changing some of your dietary habits then my advice probably won't be your cup of tea.

Let's be honest here. Along with exercise, food has virtually EVERYTHING to do with our health, our metabolism, and our weight. If you really believe you can eat pretty much whatever you want- and that it won't make a difference in terms of your health and weight- that is certainly your business and your right. In fact to this day, many doctors still tell their patients that "you can go ahead and eat whatever you like; it doesn't matter". However, America is filled to bursting with grossly overweight folks who are going through their lives doing precisely that- eating whatever they like. We have an obesity –and health- crisis going on in America today, and I-along with countless other doctors, researchers, food "gurus", ordinary folks, and others feel **strongly** that there is an unmistakable and direct link between our health and our diets.

I am not one of those who believe that our "food is out to get us" and that food has suddenly become "the enemy". I really love food- and take enormous pleasure in eating! In fact it is the pleasure that I get from healthy, great food that makes me want to share with others the joys, and the benefits from eating really wholesome, healthy food. We just need to make a clear distinction between what is truly good for us and what is not.

The real issue, from my perspective, is that way too much of the food too many Americans eat these days is of very poor quality. And frankly it is these low quality, nutrient- poor, calorie-excessive foods that are playing havoc with so many of our fellow citizen's metabolisms.

Food can be either wonderfully, powerfully nutritious, mediocre, or just plain crummy-and it is this spectrum of quality that is so important to understand. If the vast majority of our diet is powerfully nutritious, then sure, (very) occasional indulgences of mediocre or even crummy food might be ok. But if we are honest, we might find that the majority of our diet is actually quite mediocre at best and too often pretty crummy. It is this preponderance of poor quality, low-nutrient diets that needs to be reversed if we are going to turn around a nation of poorly functioning, struggling metabolisms.

As you will see in this book, the solution to eating a powerfully nutritious diet is actually common sense- and once you get the hang of it, you will see that it is also surprisingly easy- and delicious too! Unfortunately, given the onslaught of advertising and the cult of convenience that is at the heart of fast food today, such common sense just isn't that common! Instead, mostly we grab what is cheap, convenient, and filling.

Unfortunately along with cheap, convenient, and filling comes bad fats, too much salt, empty calories in the form of white flour and white sugar, and plenty of preservatives, GMOs, hormones, artificial colors and artificial flavors. What we have here is the typical picture of processed "junk foods" filled with "empty calories" and synthetic ingredients. Eating "nutrient-dense" means turning this situation around.

 What we don't have in the current picture- what in fact is too often lost or missing- is nature. Nature doesn't give us empty calories- it gives us "nutrient-dense" calories. "Empty calories" are calories from foods where the nutrients have been processed out or stripped off. The classic examples are white flour and white sugar. Nutrient-dense calories are the opposite. These are calories that are naturally accompanied by the vitamins, minerals, pigments, enzymes, fiber and other nutrients that our bodies need.

What does this have to do with the state of our metabolisms? Pretty much everything! Our metabolic pathways require – every step of the way- key vitamins or minerals to make their pathways work. If these key nutrients are in short supply, the pathways slow down or struggle. The result is a sluggish or "asleep at the wheel" metabolism that simply cannot do the job it needs to do. And a sluggish metabolism simply isn't able to burn calories efficiently. This is often the key to weight gain in most of us.

We've all heard the saying, "you are what you eat". This old cliché is actually literally true- pretty much every cell in your body is composed of the atoms and molecules that come from the foods we ingest, the water we drink, and the air we inhale. From one perspective, we are walking test tubes! Every cell in your body performs many tasks and functions, and the energy they require comes from complex metabolic pathways occurring inside special structures within the cell itself. The good news is, we know now how to optimize these pathways. And we know too what can slow them down.

You CAN lose weight. Some of us have tried- many times, with varying degrees of success. If your program had worked- permanently- you probably would not be reading these words now. Many people are to the point where they are either ready to give up, are really frustrated, or simply have lost hope or the belief and confidence that they can do it. I think this is a real shame. No one is doomed to be unhealthy or severely overweight. We are not born that way. It is not in our genes to be obese. It is simply that we are not doing what needs to be done in order to have an optimally operating metabolism. Adopting a truly nutrient-dense diet can have an amazing effect on our bodies. Your cells are waiting for you!

The Weight Loss Landscape Today

Why another book on weight loss? Hasn't everything been written and said on the subject already? Can any of the myriads of programs out there really accomplish what they promise? Does it really matter what I eat? I just put weight on no matter what I do!

These are excellent observations and questions. Why indeed yet another book on losing weight? The answer to these questions might be interesting and surprising. First let me tell you something that might shock some of you. This is *not* a book about weight loss! Well, let me clarify that. If you follow this book you can and will lose weight- in many cases quite a bit of weight (*if* you are carrying around a lot of extra pounds).

So if this isn't another "weight loss book" then what is it? The quick answer is, it is first and foremost a book about straightening out your metabolism and getting healthy. But the key point here is, **if you straighten out your metabolism and get optimally healthy, you will come into balance, and you <u>will</u> lose weight.**

The key message of this book is that your food choices matter. How is this book different from the many other "diet" books out there? Most diet books and programs talk a lot about how *much* to eat (or not to eat). They teach and promote counting calories and grams of fat, carbs, etc. You might be relieved to know that in *The Nutrient-Dense Diet* there is no math! You will never ever be asked to count a single calorie or gram of anything! This book is different because it is about quality- not amounts. This may come as a shock, but the *amount* of what you eat doesn't matter that much- it's *what* you eat that matters- not *how much* you eat. Don't believe me? There are plenty of thin people out there who eat a lot more calories than their more overweight peers. The difference is in their metabolisms. And that is what this book is all about- helping you with your metabolism.

Losing weight depends upon you. I can't do it for you, nor can any doctor or weight loss "specialist". This is the key missing piece- your motivation. If you are willing to really "go for it" then you can achieve wonders. If you are ambivalent or full of self-doubt and hesitancy, then the best plan in the world will probably not work- not because of any flaw in the program, but because you will probably not have the will power or ambition to see it through.

The "Nutrient-Smart" program works. In fact it works perfectly, safely, naturally, and effectively. But- it only works if it is applied. I have taught nutrition to thousands of individuals. What I have discovered is that there is a real spectrum among people in terms of motivation, will power, and enthusiasm. The truth is, many people get "stuck", and it isn't just their metabolism that is stuck. We all fall into habits, and we all have a tendency to get complacent. Many of us decide it is easier to just "stay the course" and continue to do what we have been doing. Even if it means our health isn't that great and our bodies are getting older, saggier, and heavier we often feel that we should just accept it. It's just too much trouble, too much "work" to change or to try and reverse nature or the aging process. And for many of us, our attachment to our eating lifestyle is so entrenched that we simply won't consider making changes even if it means continuing on a path that leads inevitably to poor health, low energy, and a reduced quality of life.

This is the "darker side" of a slowed down metabolism. It seems a slow metabolism doesn't just slow us down biochemically- it might also slow down our enthusiasm, zest for life, self-confidence and motivation as well. Some people with weight issues also experience mild depression as well. A slow metabolism isn't selective- our brains and nervous system rely on metabolic energy as well as all the other tissues of our body.

When I teach or give a lecture on some aspect of nutrition or weight loss, I often start out by saying that nutrition is about self-esteem, self-worth, and a sense of dignity. This is not what we normally expect to hear when we learn about nutrition, but I think this is actually the perfect starting point. **We need to really believe we are worthwhile, and that we deserve to have a healthy, energetic, vibrant body and health.** If we don't believe this deep down, then we are probably defeated before we even begin!

Our belief systems matter! What we say to ourselves and how we view ourselves is crucial to the type of life we live. If we subtly don't really value ourselves or don't think we are worthy or deserving of having a healthy body then we very likely are not going to put the effort into trying to have one. On the other hand, if we really want a healthy body and feel that we are deserving of one, then we will be much more likely to do whatever it takes to get there.

There are many different diets and "eating philosophies" around today. Recent best sellers have advocated eating more carbs, or fewer carbs; diets very high in protein, and some that are very low in protein. There are raw diets, cooked diets, "Zone^{tm}" diets and "South Beach^{tm}" diets in addition to gluten-free diets, "Paleo" diets, The Blood Type Diet^{tm} and more. How is "The Nutrient-Dense" diet different? Well, to begin with, "The Nutrient-Dense Diet" isn't really a diet at all- it's an eating lifestyle. And surprisingly, it has a lot in common with the best of virtually all of the above-mentioned diets.

As I just said, The Nutrient-Dense Diet isn't really a diet at all in the classic sense of the word. Adopting a nutrient-smart way of eating simply means one thing- paying attention to the *quality* of what we eat. It might surprise you but eating nutrient-smart has nothing to do with counting calories- or grams of fat or carbs. Instead the focus is on eating fresh, mostly unprocessed nutritious foods- and largely avoiding foods that aren't nutrient-dense or ones that contribute metabolic "road blocks".

Changing *what* we eat actually changes the *environment* within our bodies, and in particular within our cells. Just as animals and plants have to adapt (or face the consequences) to changes in their environments, so to do our cells, tissues, and organs. This is the crux of the cliché, "we are what we eat", and it is the crux too of "The Nutrient-Smart Weight Loss Program".

Medical research has discovered so much in recent decades. One of the many exciting and promising areas is our understanding that the aggressiveness of cancerous cells can be altered by changing their cellular environment. Not very long ago the medical establishment believed that the environment that cancer cells grow in doesn't matter. Now the same establishment is embracing the idea that changing the cellular environment can have profound implications in cancer treatment and therapy. And this is not just true of cancer. The "cellular environment" matters in most, if not all diseases- a lot!

In a similar way, we now understand that the foods we choose can have profound implications for the quality of the inner environment of our bodies and cells. And as we have seen, it is the ability of our food to supply the key nutrients that fuel the metabolic pathways within our cells that determines the quality of our metabolic pathways. That is the nutrient-dense insight and the nutrient-dense edge!

If "we are what we eat" then it stands to reason that eating junk foods full of dead, empty calories, will lead inevitably to a junky, unhealthy body. But what if the opposite is true? Could eating vibrant, healthy, energy and nutrient-rich foods lead to a more vibrant, energetic and healthier body? The evidence overwhelmingly says, yes! This is eating nutrient-smart!

Part I

The Metabolic Puzzle

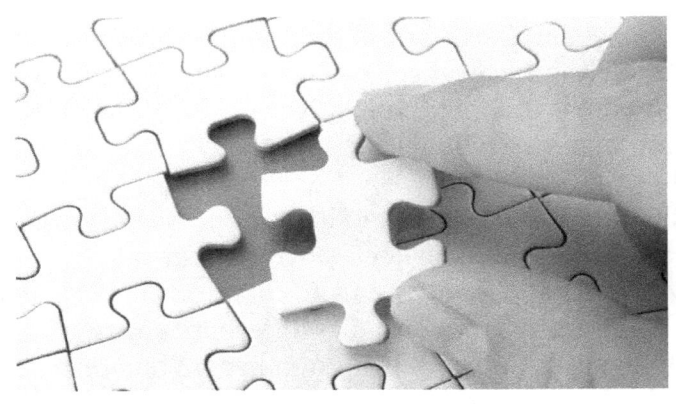

Chapter 1

The Metabolic Puzzle

The key to effective weight loss is solving the metabolic puzzle. Our metabolism is central to understanding why we gain weight, and is quite often the principle difference between overweight and normal weight individuals. If we are going to understand how to work with our bodies in healthier ways, we simply have to understand what and how our metabolism works. Fortunately, our metabolism is not something we are stuck with- it can be improved and optimized! This is the heart of our approach to weight loss. The old idea that weight gain is due to too many calories is simplistic and obsolete. The metabolic puzzle presents a new and modern understanding that more accurately reflects the reality that is going on in our bodies.

"Metabolism" is the word we use to describe the essence of living things. It is a neat word that summarizes the many different chemical processes and reactions within our cells and bodies. To put it simply, "metabolism" is the difference between an elephant, flea, bird, or human on the one hand, and a rock on the other hand. Living things have a metabolism; non-living things (like rocks) do not. To say it another way, living things are alive because they have countless metabolic reactions going on constantly within every cell, which keeps them alive. When something dies, its metabolism stops, very quickly - as the various metabolic reactions come to a halt.

Obviously a subject such as metabolism can be very complicated- it is an enormous job to keep an organism alive, with all its specialized cells and structures and functions and needs. In fact, there are literally millions of different chemical reactions occurring every moment during our lives. Your brain functions in ways that are very different from the demands and activities of a muscle cell in your arm or a cell in your kidney or pancreas. But all of the different cells, tissues, and organs within us require one thing in common- energy. Without a steady reliable source of biologically available energy to power these metabolic reactions, our cells would immediately grind to a halt, like pulling the plug from an appliance. So how- and where- do we get this energy from?

Making Cellular Energy

Cellular energy is something every cell produces. This is the miracle of life. We breathe air and ingest water and food for nutrients-which are the chemical raw materials for our metabolisms. And our cells do the rest. It is quite amazing- each cell knows precisely what to do and how to do it, no matter how complicated or specialized the task. Whether it is manufacturing insulin from special pancreatic cells, or producing thyroid hormones from within our thyroid gland or producing anti- stress hormones in our adrenal glands or making neurotransmitters so the nerve cells in our brain can talk to each other or signals telling our bone marrow to make red and white blood cells in the right quantities and proportions, our cells work ceaselessly. And all require a constant supply of energy and raw materials.

Special instructional "guide books" or "user manuals" within parts of every cell direct the show- making very few mistakes. These instructions come from our inherited genetic legacy- our DNA and RNA, unique molecules which reside in the nuclei of each of our trillions of cells, and these mega molecules act as architect, foreman and project supervisor all in one. When they do their job properly and give the right instructions and all the necessary raw materials are handy, then things tend to go very well and the result is a healthy functioning organism. Of course sometimes things don't go exactly according to plan, and the result can be sub optimal health or disease.

So in summary, our metabolism is the totality of myriads of life-sustaining chemical reactions that occur within each of the cells of living organisms- both plant and animal. These reactions generate the energy and produce the molecules needed for living things to grow, repair, reproduce, and regulate themselves.

If you took biology in High School or college, then you might have learned that the "currency" of energy in the body is a molecule called ATP. ATP (adenosine triphosphate) is the storehouse or "holder" of energy in the form of high-energy chemical bonds that are used to drive chemical reactions. ATP production therefore, is the "goal" of the most fundamental metabolic processes within the cell- making ATP is what living cells do. Stop making ATP, and the cell (and organism) dies.

The process of manufacturing ATP occurs in specialized structures within the cell, called "mitochondria". Scientists often refer to mitochondria as the batteries or energy factories of the cell because this is where energy- in the form of ATP- is "made". Mitochondria are sensitive structures, and they require specific nutrients in order to do their jobs effectively. As we will see, we can use this knowledge to our advantage if we want to support energy production in the body. The mitochondria are also where fats and carbohydrates are "burned" or combusted and converted into energy. Metabolically speaking, the mitochondria are "ground zero" for energy production.

The process of energy production is well known in biology and is sometimes referred to as "cellular respiration" because it usually takes place in the presence of oxygen. But don't confuse this with ordinary breathing. Cellular respiration and energy production actually has to do with 'electron transfer' mechanisms and other complicated biochemical chain reactions. The key to a healthy metabolism is having healthy cellular respiration going on.

But this is also the Achilles heel of health too- and poor nutrition, a lack of key nutrients, or the presence of metabolic toxins and other interferences can stifle or suffocate this process, leading to a metabolic slowing down and consequently, weight gain. The purpose of this book is to show you how to take the clamps off your cells and optimize cellular respiration so you can operate at peak efficiency.

Producing ATP is vital for us to be alive and to function well. It is said that we produce our own weight in ATP molecules every day, which is quite an astounding statistic if you think about it! ATP fuels literally every single chemical reaction in our body- it is the common thread that unifies the myriads of diverse biochemical activities in every cell, tissue, and organ within us. It is like the current that comes into our houses and supplies every appliance, outlet, and fixture in our home with the same type of electricity.

Most of these cellular biochemical processes end up creating specific proteins that our bodies need. Proteins are assembled according to our cell's unique blueprints, in the DNA and RNA within the cell's nuclei. Hormones, neurotransmitters, muscle tissue, hemoglobin, connective tissues such as collagen or keratin (which is what your hair is made from), and many other molecules are all examples of such proteins. Our metabolism governs whether we do this efficiently and effectively, or whether it is a struggle and challenge. The overall state of our metabolism also governs our body weight and percentage of body fat, and whether we feel energetic, vibrantly alive, and creative, or whether we feel lethargic, sluggish and even depressed or unmotivated. Improving and optimizing our metabolic situation is the heart of an effective weight management program- and is vitally important for our overall health as well.

So how do we use this basic understanding to our own individual advantage to solve our personal metabolic puzzle? Let's explore this a bit more. Fortunately, the answer is simpler and closer at hand than you may think!

Despite the fear you may have felt at the idea of chemistry class, most chemical reactions are fairly straightforward. Usually to create something, say protein "F", we go in simple, small steps, from A to B to C to D to E to F. To get from say, B to C, we may need certain conditions or elements or compounds. To then get from C to D, we may need an entirely different set of elements. Amazingly, these chain reactions occur all the time, hundreds of millions of times every second. Yet sometimes our cells struggle, or have to cope with roadblocks and challenges that we put in their way. So what are these roadblocks and what can we do to remove them?

First of all, how do we get from A to B or E to F? In the human body biochemical reactions are usually mediated by compounds called co-enzymes. Co-enzymes are molecules that act as chemical catalysts or facilitators of chemical reactions. Most of the time catalysts are specific vitamins or minerals. This is the basis of the science of nutrition. Vitamins and minerals are essentially the lubricants that grease the engine of our metabolic reactions. If your car engine runs out of oil it will seize up. If our cells run out of vitamins or minerals, our metabolic reactions will likewise struggle, and then grind to a halt. We call such minerals and vitamins "essential" for this simple reason. We have to have them to stay alive. They are "essential" because our body cannot manufacture them- they have to come from our diets.

When we think of "nutrition" many of us have been conditioned to think primarily of three things- proteins, fats, and carbohydrates. And it is true that these are the major building blocks of the body- in fact we call these the "macro-nutrients" because we require all three of these classes of nutrients in relatively large quantities. However when we speak about cellular nutrition and cellular metabolic pathways, it is the nutrients we require in comparatively smaller amounts – the minerals and vitamins- that are just as vital, if not more so. These "micro-nutrients" are the heart of nutrient-dense eating and metabolic optimization. And even though we require these nutrients in relatively small amounts, many of us are not getting what is required to keep our metabolic engines humming along efficiently. And this is a big piece of the metabolic puzzle that is leading to much of the obesity problem (among others) in the world today.

Empty Calories

It turns out that processing food tends to remove most of these naturally occurring vitamins and minerals. The truth is, most packaged, convenient, "fast food" and "junk" foods these days have had much of their original micro-nutrient content stripped away. So called "fortification" of food puts back a handful of vitamins and some minerals, but the vitamins are synthetic, less effective versions of the original, and much of what is removed can never be replaced. The result is that much of what people eat these days is nutrient deficient. The calories are still there- sometimes more so- but the nutrient levels are diminished, often dramatically. The most obvious examples of empty calorie, nutrient-deficient foods are the two that are most commonly consumed- white sugar and white flour.

We call these "empty calorie" foods, as both sugar and flour contribute calories, but are empty – or nearly so- of any vitamins or minerals. As such, neither can provide the important trace nutrients necessary for our metabolic chain reactions. And it is obvious that excess consumption of both can contribute to weight gain, poor health, and obesity.

Unfortunately, too many of us rely on too many "empty calorie" foods as a prominent part of our diets. Eating too many carb heavy foods and consuming a relatively large percentage of our calories in the form of breads, cakes, cookies, pizza, bagels, English muffins, buns, toaster pastries, muffins, and many other foods is a big reason behind the weight problem in America today. Add to these white flour foods our love affair with sugar in all manner of foods and beverages, and it becomes clear that we are feeding ourselves way too many empty calories. Losing weight simply has to address this imbalanced ratio of too many calories and not enough (micro) nutrients. Fortunately there is a simple, healthy, and delicious solution to this pervasive problem!

The Nutrient-Dense Solution

The opposite of empty calories are "nutrient-dense" calories, and they are everywhere. Much of the remainder of this book will be an in-depth look at nutrient-dense foods- what they are, how to find them, and how to enjoy them. As you will see, nutrient-dense eating is really a return to "common sense" eating, and is a much more natural and sensible way of eating than the fast food mentality that has taken over our convenience- oriented world. Eating nutrient-dense is eating nutrient-smart!

Eating healthy and returning to some basics is both necessary and empowering, and once you try it- satisfying- and easy too! If you want to lose weight, regain your health and zest for life, then there is really no other way. Millions of people eat this way, and so can you! And it is easier than you think.

Like all things, there are two sides to the metabolic puzzle. Some things, like the right vitamins and minerals (and some other key nutrients) are metabolic facilitators which we need while other things operate as metabolic poisons which we should obviously avoid. If we are to have an optimally functioning metabolism, it just makes sense to seek out and do the right things to promote healthy metabolic functioning and avoid the things that are toxic or metabolic poisons. Fortunately science has learned a lot about what can adversely affect our metabolisms.

Some Common Metabolic Toxins

Scientists often use such knowledge for specific purposes. For example, many of the most commonly used insecticides and pesticides today work by literally poisoning or shutting down certain metabolic pathways in insects, so their respiration, or nervous systems are inoperable. Now we are certainly not insects, but we do share some of the same enzyme systems with our buggy friends. Perhaps this is one of many reasons why organically grown foods might be better for us. Cutting back on the load of agricultural chemicals that we incidentally ingest along with most conventionally grown food might be one piece of the puzzle for lightening the load on our overstressed metabolisms.

Other commonly known metabolic poisons include chlorine and mercury. Mercury is highly toxic to our nervous system, and is widely considered to be one of the very most toxic substances known. Certain fish, such as shark, swordfish, and tuna unfortunately contain higher levels of mercury, and are probably best avoided, especially for women who might get pregnant-high mercury levels in mother's milk can be a risk factor for the developing brain and nervous system of her offspring. And chlorine, of course, is ever-present in almost all of the beverages and water that we drink as well as the water we bathe and shower in.

However, the most common and most significant metabolic toxins in the normal American diet (sometimes referred to as the Standard American Diet, or SAD for short) **are synthetic hormones, and damaged oils**. Let's take a moment and briefly discuss each of these.

Synthetic hormones are bio-engineered hormone "look-alikes" that the animal food industry uses extensively to fatten their livestock and to speed up the time for their sexual maturation, all so they can grow bigger and fatter and be killed quicker and turned into profit faster. Commercial chickens (and their eggs), all pork products, beef, and dairy animals are all raised this way these days. Except for certified organically raised, free range animals, you can be pretty sure that all of the hamburgers, bacon, chicken wings, cheese, ice cream, ham, steaks, pepperonis on your pizza and so much else come loaded with biologically active hormones- that you ingest. Since these synthetic estrogens and related compounds are used to fatten up animals, doesn't it make sense that they could contribute to our weight gain as well? Why take a chance? **If your goal is to really lose weight, then I *strongly* emphasize eliminating *all* non-organic commercial sources of animal meat, eggs, and dairy.** This step alone can make an enormous difference.

Synthetic hormones fool and confuse our own metabolic biochemistry and as such are considered to be metabolic poisons. The vast majority of Americans eat diets that are primarily composed of such agribusiness raised meat- pretty much all fast food chains and major restaurants *only* serve this kind of meat and dairy. Is it any wonder we have an epidemic of overweight people in our country? From the milk we have on our cereal for breakfast (or in our coffee) to the burger at lunch to the chicken or pizza we have for dinner to the ice cream we have for dessert our meals tend to be loaded with synthetic hormones. In addition, many researchers strongly believe that these synthetic hormones may be carcinogenic as well. Please avoid these foods if you are sincere about regaining your health and your body!

Fats and Oils –Our Friends and Foes

The other class of foods that are strongly "anti-metabolism" are the wrong kinds of fats and oils. Good fats are actually wonderful and very important sources of healthful nutrients, and we will discuss their beneficial role in actually boosting our metabolism and helping us lose weight in a following chapter. **But unfortunately, most of the fats and oils we ingest in the SAD (Standard American Diet) are the wrong kind- and act as powerful inhibitors of our metabolism.** Let's explore why.

Good fats and oils are essential for building healthy membranes within our cells, and for other important reasons as well. We don't commonly think of fats as "good guys" but in reality, the right ones are extremely important for optimal health. But since "we are what we eat" if bad fats are all that are available, the body will use them wherever it needs to employ them.

Where do we use fats and oils (collectively called, "lipids") in our body? One of the most important places is within our cell's membranes. Cell membranes are actually crucial structures and their role in maintaining and fostering health is finally being well understood. Membranes contain portals- the "doorways" and windows into a cell- and it is through them that nutrients are allowed to enter and waste products (toxins) exit. The precise shape and functioning of these doors and windows is a result of special properties imparted by the flexibility and shape of the fat molecules. When the right fat molecules are used as building blocks, the doors can do their job efficiently. But when the wrong fats are used, difficulties can arise, making it harder for nutrients to get in and for wastes to exit. This is bad news for the cells, and bad news for us!

Remember the mitochondria and the ATP molecules that they produce via "cellular respiration"? Mitochondria have membranes of their own, and guess what- they are made principally of fatty acids, just like "regular" cell membranes. Applying the principle of "we are what we eat", we can see that

24

eating fried, rancid, damaged, or trans-fats can result in these oils being incorporated into the mitochondrial membranes. This can start to literally "gum up the works" and reduce the ability of these structures to produce adequate or optimal levels of ATP, slowing down cellular respiration and lowering overall energy production. So, energy goes down, calories aren't used, fat gets stored and we get tired and gain weight. Sound familiar?

What are the good fats and which are the bad ones? Good fats are naturally occurring, minimally processed oils, such as from avocados, olives, non-rancid nuts and seeds, grass fed organic butter, good fresh fish oils, coconut oil, hemp oil and flax oils. These are all healthy nutrient-dense oils that can support and aid a struggling metabolism. These are the "nutrient-smart" choices.

On the other hand, the vast majority of oils that Americans eat these days are incorporated into much of the fast foods we eat. Heavily processed and sterilized oils such as canola, soybean, corn, cottonseed, and peanut oils are all commonly used by the food industries. They are cheap, but they are certainly not nutritious. By the time they end up on the shelf or in our food they are a far cry from their natural state. And most if not all, have now been genetically modified as well. Another problem with these oils is that they contain mainly what are called "omega-6" fats, which are pro-inflammatory fatty acids. Inflammation in excess anywhere is not good, and within our cells is yet another major cause of metabolic malfunctioning.

The other problem with most of these oils is that they often are highly heated, which can alter their chemical structure and lead to toxic by-products including free radicals. Free radicals are highly energetic "unbalanced" molecules that tend to attack nearby atoms and molecules as they search for available electrons, leading to damage, inflammation, and breakdown.

Since these oils are incorporated into important and highly sensitive parts like cell membranes, I strongly urge you to avoid them if your goal is to be healthy and to lose weight. If you have a bottle of such oil in your pantry, I recommend you toss it out! Many home recipes such as pancakes or muffins call for a little oil so these bad oils tend to be used more commonly than most of us realize. My advice is: toss out the old oil from your pantry and use a new jar of coconut oil instead for your frying, sautéing or baking!

Frying of course is the cooking technique of applying extremely high temperatures to fats and oils, which can molecularly damage and alter their structures leading to further free-radical generation. Fried foods are never healthy, and do no good at all for your body. Scientists now believe that much of the epidemic of arteriosclerosis (hardened arteries) and cardiovascular disease that we are experiencing is due in part to these fried fats and oils being deposited along the inner linings of our arteries. French fries, potato and corn chips, and fried chicken and similar foods should not be considered healthy foods by any stretch of the imagination, and can definitely be linked to altered, struggling metabolic functioning, weight gain, heart disease and other serious health problems.

Getting Unstuck

We really are miracles of nature. Our metabolic reactions are highly complex, intricate and finely tuned processes that are meant to work together like instruments in an orchestra to create a beautiful outcome- the gift of health and the ability for us to be creative, happy individuals. However, eating unnatural foods that are highly processed, nutrient-depleted, and full of metabolic poisons such as pesticides and synthetic hormone residues can "gum up the works"- slowing down our metabolic processes and leading to lowered energy and poor health. Cells that have compromised membranes may have difficulty shuttling nutrients in and wastes out. Such a situation can cause a slowing of the ability of cells to "burn" calories for energy; as a result we may start to slow down ourselves, feeling tired, uninspired, and even mentally depressed or defeated. Instead of burning calories and liberating energy, calories essentially turn to fat, and become "storage depots" for a rainy day.

I call this situation "cellular dormancy" because the cells struggle, slow down, and seemingly start to go to sleep. This is what happens when we see quite obese people- their cells have gone into metabolic hibernation. They still function, but at a reduced level of effectiveness- it is like when your computer is in sleep mode. Energy is being conserved: the computer is still "on", but it is not expending energy to perform its normal functions. In such people, their metabolism is likewise powered down: so they gain weight, they lack energy, and their health is at risk. What this book is about is "waking up cellular dormancy." The good news is that a dormant or sleepy metabolism can be woken up- it can become "unstuck".

To be honest, many people are quite "stuck" in their eating habits as well. People get into routines- of habit and convenience mostly- and when confronted with the idea of change, often a lot of resistance can arise. But the good news is that we are never as "stuck" as we may think we are. If you truly want to lose weight, or regain your health, or just feel better you can. It really all comes down to motivation- and believing in yourself.

Most people don't lose much of their excess weight- not because they cannot, but because they have talked themselves out of it before they even have started! People come up with all sorts of excuses: "I don't have time to eat healthy", "It's too much work", "My husband (or kids) won't go along with it", "I don't like health food", "I'm too busy", I've tried it and it didn't work", "I can't afford it", etc. etc.

The truth is, anyone can lose weight- the question is, do you *really* want to? I encounter people every day who say they want to lose weight, but when it comes down to doing what it takes, they quickly back down or give up. I think this is really sad, because losing weight is actually easy, and feeling good sure beats feeling crummy. But as we said, people get used to being a certain way, and feeling a certain way. We have an obesity epidemic in this country- there are way more overweight and grossly overweight (obese) people today than any time in history, so clearly many people are in this situation. The sad thing is, it simply doesn't need to be this way. In the following chapters I will show you exactly how to improve your metabolism through eating nutrient-dense foods and how to jump-start a really stuck metabolism through the use of some safe, natural supplements and of course, some sensible exercise. This program works- I guarantee it- but it has to be put into practice. That part is up to you.

Addictive Foods

There is another, darker part of the weight loss story that most of us never think about. Many people sincerely want to lose weight, but don't realize they are battling another demon- addiction. Typically we think of certain substances like cigarettes or drugs as addictive. What we don't commonly know is that we are quite often addicted- literally- to much of what we eat as well.

Food scientists and food companies have done a great job at getting us to buy their products. Ever wonder why you "crave" certain foods? Well the answer is quite often in the "secret sauce"! Food flavors in particular are often highly addictive thanks to the molecules used to create them. In particular MSG (monosodium glutamate) and its relatives are highly addictive molecules that work with the brain and nervous system to trick us into perceiving flavor and intensity that is not really there. Once we get used to these flavors and intense tastes, our brains literally crave them and expect them to be there.

Another highly addictive molecule is Aspartame, or "NutraSweet", the artificial sweetener. And for many, a protein in milk known as casein is also an addictive molecule. If you eat a lot of dairy or processed foods or fast foods then chances are you consume a lot of these kinds of molecules. And if you tend to crave certain foods, brands, and restaurant chains and you have a hard time giving up your "comfort foods" and brands for less processed, more natural foods, then there is a good chance you are literally "addicted" to these tastes. You can break these addictions- but like all addictions, it is never easy or simple. However, realizing what you are dealing with is a big step forward!

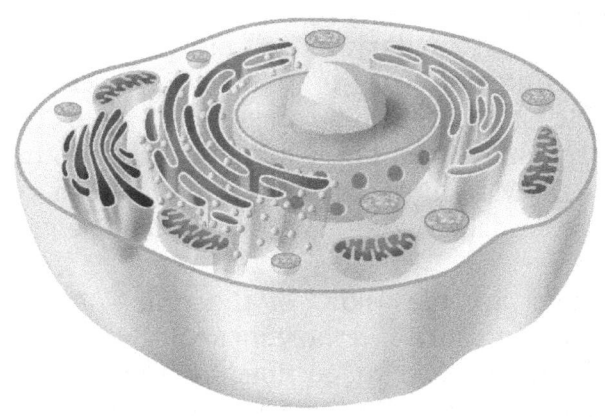

Chapter 2

The Cell: Metabolism's Ground Zero

We are made of cells-trillions of them. Most are invisible to the eye- they are far too small to see without a microscope- but some, such as certain nerve cells, actually can extend for several feet. Cells make up nervous tissue, our skin, the linings of our lungs and intestines, the muscle that is our heart, our various organs and glands, our bones, and even the immune- enforcing white cells in our lymph and blood. Despite their common origins and common genetic inheritances, cells differentiate into an amazing array of shapes, functions, and roles.

Despite their apparent differences, virtually all cells have several things in common; and some of these have an enormous impact on cellular functioning, overall efficiency, and metabolism. Understanding the basics of how our cells work is crucial to understanding our metabolism- the underlying basis of our health.

For one thing, most cells share several common structures, such as their outermost boundary, or cell membrane. Also, virtually all cells have mitochondria- the sub- cellular energy factories where the nitty-gritty of cellular metabolism takes place. These structures are where most of the actual energy production takes place. But the key to understanding mitochondria, metabolism, and cells in general, lies in understanding their membranes.

Cell membranes are the "skin" of the cell. They also contain portals for the transport of important molecules into and out of the cells. Nutrients need to be able to freely enter the cell's interior, where they can be incorporated into new structures, replace worn out ones, be used for the creation of energy, and mediate other biochemical reactions. At the same time, metabolic waste products, such as CO_2 and urea must be able to readily exit the cell so that they can be carried away, to be exhaled, sweated, or urinated out of the body. If for some reason they can't leave, they may build up within the cell, like an overflowing landfill or toxic waste site. Metabolic slowing or poisoning may be the inevitable result. It is easy to see that the integrity and functional efficiency of cell membranes is crucial to maintaining cellular health.

We have already quoted the famous saying, "you are what you eat." This statement naturally extends to our cells as well. In other words, our cells are made from what we eat. Our cells' membranes are a great example of this. Comprised mainly of a unique combination of proteins and lipids (nutritionally derived fats and/or oils), the key characteristics of cell membranes such as their fluidity or suppleness as well as the size and efficiency of the "windows" or portals embedded in the membrane depends upon the quality and type of fatty acids that are incorporated into the membrane's structure. Like a well-greased revolving door or an easy to open and shut window, our membranes need to be soft, pliable and lubricated.

Scientists have shown that eating a diet rich in trans-fats (from hydrogenated oils), found in relatively large amounts in processed foods in the Standard American Diet, or SAD, can impede the functioning of cell membranes. By altering the shape and characteristics of the portals in the cell membranes, trans-fats may in fact slow down the rates with which nutrients can enter and wastes can leave the cell. Mitochondrial membranes are similarly at risk. A nutrient-dense diet, on the other hand, by supplying a larger percentage of healthful essential fatty acids, can help ensure healthy cell and mitochondrial membranes, which will improve overall metabolic functioning and efficiency.

Another exciting area of research involves the influence of different diets and foods on our genes (for more information, see chapter on "Food as Information"). **What this really means is that what we eat actually communicates or "talks" to our DNA.** As it turns out, specific molecules and nutrients in food actually influence the expression of individual genes. In turn the genes in our cells (and in the mitochondria as well) code for the production of specific proteins. This indicates that the signals we send into our bodies can intimately affect our health and welfare on a more subtle level than we ever suspected. To put it another way: components in our food can actually turn genes on and off! In this way we can see once again the profound truth that "we are what we eat". Obviously our food choices do *matter-* in ways that are subtle, profound, and significant.

This understanding of the role of food in ensuring the health and optimal functioning of our cells, tissues, and organs is at the forefront of the modern science of nutrition. Cell physiology (physiology is the science and study of how the body actually *functions*) is making rapid strides, much of which will continue to shed light on overall metabolic activities and its consequences for our health and wellbeing.

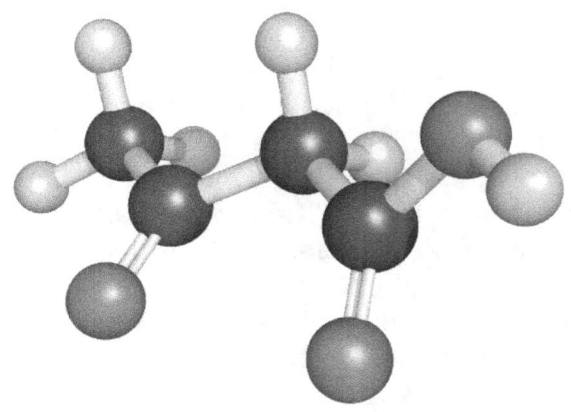

Chapter 3

Understanding Metabolism: How Our Cells Make Energy

Simply stated, the word "metabolism" refers to the sum total of the large group of processes that take place at the cellular level. Turning food into the energy that is used to fuel all of the many biochemical reactions that are necessary for life to occur is the basis of staying alive. Cell division, tissue repair, synthesis of hormones and other bio-molecules, movement, muscle contraction, respiration, digestion, and nerve conduction are just some of the tasks that require a constant supply of "energy" in order to take place. Without an intact and functioning metabolism, life simply could not exist.

Lifestyle, genetics, environmental factors, stress and other mental states, the thyroid gland and other organ systems, medications, and many other influences all affect our overall metabolic efficiency. Understanding the basics of metabolic functioning can help you make sense out of the important roles that different foods in our diet can play in our bodies.

Energy is produced in our bodies in a highly specific way- through complex chemical reactions that are tightly orchestrated and well-coordinated. This series of biochemical steps are collectively known as the "Citric Acid Cycle", and are also sometimes referred to as the "Krebs Cycle" after one of its key discoverers. One of the principle end results of the citric acid cycle is the production of energy- packaged for use by our cells in the form of a highly energetic molecule called ATP (short for Adenosine Tri-Phosphate). This entire process occurs in uniquely specialized structures within each cell, called mitochondria. Essentially, mitochondria can be thought of as tiny but efficient factories that are responsible for the production of ATP- those energy-storing molecules necessary for life's many activities.

ATP is ultimately generated in the citric acid cycle from our food-which is one of the main purposes of eating- to supply the raw materials for energy production. Food is also necessary to supply additional essential substances such as vitamins and minerals-which are necessary for the choreography of literally thousands of other biochemical reactions to occur. Nutrient deficiencies or shortages can dramatically alter our body's functioning by pulling the plug on some of these reactions. Poor health, lowered energy, and an altered metabolism can all result from key nutrient deprivations.

The usual main fuel source for driving the citric acid cycle forward and ultimately producing ATP molecules are carbohydrates. Carbohydrates- sugars and starches- are broken down by certain enzymes into smaller molecules that are ultimately shuttled into the mitochondrial factories where the citric acid cycle can do its thing.
But carbohydrates are not the only fuel source for the citric acid cycle. When carbohydrates are in limited supply such as during a fast, starvation, or in cases of extreme endurance events, the

body can also make use of dietary or stored proteins and also fats as fuel for the Krebs cycle. This is a far less efficient way to produce energy, but nonetheless it is an important and useful back-up plan. However, as we will see, in some people this can lead to other health consequences.

The important factors in metabolic efficiency then, are the relative availability of the different classes of foods (carbohydrates, fats and proteins), the presence or absence of specific nutrients such as vitamins and minerals, the activity and influence of certain hormones in our bodies, and the role of other contributing influences such as environmental toxins, cellular poisons, and others. Clearly our metabolisms are vulnerable to a host of influences, both positive and negative.

The Nutrient-Dense Diet is designed to maximize overall metabolic efficiency by (1) supplying higher levels of trace minerals, vitamins, and other nutrients that are necessary for the enzymes involved in the citric acid cycle to do their part, and (2) decreasing the load of unnecessary food additives and other metabolic poisons- substances that may depress or slow down metabolic functioning. Both of these contributions are made through adopting a more nutrient-dense way of eating. In addition, a nutrient-dense diet lower in refined carbohydrates might help your metabolism through lessening insulin secretion and improving the responsiveness of your cells to the insulin that is available. "Insulin insensitivity" is an important factor in many cases of weight gain and metabolic inefficiency.

There are lots of ways to send messages to your "metabolic self"- messages that can signal it to either slow down or speed up. Unfortunately, today there are far too many of the "slow down!" signals such as the repeated ingestion of synthetic estrogenic hormones from the dairy, poultry, beef, and pork industries, empty calorie snacks and junk foods, fluoride from our water and toothpaste, and many, many others. Even skipping breakfast can send the wrong message to our cells; not eating can be seen as a sign of potential starvation so the body tends to hoard its

37

calories. By not eating, we may tell our metabolism to slow down even more, so that it conserves what it gets rather than burning it for energy. Weight gain is often nature's evolutionary strategy to insure long-term survival.

In future chapters we will explore in greater depth several strategies that you can easily implement in order to "up-regulate" the metabolic machinery in your cell's mitochondria.

Chapter 4

Giving Your Mitochondria
A Helping Hand

As I mentioned, within each cell are thousands of tiny units where our cellular energy is actually made. Called "mitochondria", these cellular batteries are where our metabolism occurs. This is 'ground zero' for our health and metabolism- the place where it all happens. A lot of very technical research has focused on these organelles, and we now understand in great detail how mitochondria function, what they need to stay healthy, and what can make them struggle.

This is incredibly valuable information for us if we really want to 'take the bull by the horns' and be more proactive about our health- and our weight. This is truly exciting news- in fact this is the cutting edge of modern medicine, health, and nutrition because it shows us ways we can directly get involved with our most intimate biochemical functioning and therefore gives us the knowledge and power to take more control over our lives.

This is the heart of our metabolism - the Krebs Cycle, or as it is also known, the Citric Acid Cycle. Another closely related metabolic biochemical reaction- something known as oxidative phosphorylation, or, the electron transport chain- takes place here too. So, without getting too technical (metabolism is a very complicated process!) let's touch on some of the most important things you can do to give your mitochondria a helping hand. After all, they work hard to help us and keep us alive; shouldn't we do everything in our power to help them back? **Counteracting cellular dormancy usually really means counteracting mitochondrial inefficiency**.

The big buzz these days in holistic and nutritional circles is about free radicals, antioxidants, and something called "oxidative stress". To put it simply, the "problem" is oxidation or oxidative stress, the culprits or "bad guys" are the free radicals, and the solution or "good guys" are the antioxidants. It turns out mitochondria are particularly vulnerable to oxidative stress, and much research involving aging, disease, and metabolic problems of all sorts is zeroed in on exactly this area. Supporting our metabolic and mitochondrial health are intimately related.

As it turns out, free radicals tend to target vulnerable spots in our cells that are electron and lipid (oils) rich, and that is exactly what the mitochondria are- lipid rich sitting ducks within each cell and therefore vulnerable targets. For this reason, anti-aging research suggests that we should try to protect our mitochondria with a variety of nutritional supports, including antioxidants. Good examples of such protective antioxidants include certain vitamins, such as oil-soluble vitamin E. Natural vitamin E (not synthetic) is likely a key means to support the challenges that lipid-rich mitochondrial membranes face.

Another important antioxidant that research suggests could be helpful includes Vitamin C (ascorbic acid) and its accompanying bioflavonoids, found in abundance in most fresh fruits. Resveratrol is a substance found in red grape skins (hence found in red wine) and is a new and increasingly popular antioxidant supplement that is supported by much research. Another exciting nutrient is alpha-lipoic acid. Lipoic acid may be of particular benefit as it is unusual in that it offers dual protection for both fat and water soluble molecules. Finally, another very important group of protective antioxidants are molecules collectively known as polyphenols or flavonoids. These are molecules often associated with both cocoa solids and brightly colored fruits- such as the bright purple, red, and blue pigments associated with blueberries, raspberries, and other berries and fruits. Eating these fruits (and a little bit of dark chocolate) are delicious ways to help protect our vulnerable cellular structures!

Probably one of the biggest threats to our mitochondria comes from refined, processed fats and oils in our diet. As mentioned, mitochondrial structures contain a lot of lipid rich components. Applying the concept of "you are what you eat", we can see that eating damaged oils, such as highly heated ("oxidized"), processed oils is not a very good idea. Our national love affair with fried foods as well as the food industry's past 75 year history of extensively and increasingly using trans-fats (partially hydrogenated vegetable oils) has frankly wrecked-havoc on our cellular and mitochondrial membranes with dire consequences for our nation's health.

Fortunately we can turn this situation around. Applying the same principles that we have talked about throughout this book, we can change our membranes and other cellular structures with the right foods and nutrients. Slowly but surely, we can replace old cells, tissues, and membranes with healthier, fresher ones. Changing the *quality* of the fats and oils we eat can make a world of difference- in how we feel, how we look, and even how we age. If you are substantially overweight and looking to lose weight, one of the most important starting points will be to do a complete "makeover" in terms of the fats and oils you use on a daily basis.

So what are the good, healthy, tissue-building fats? Fortunately there are plenty. I recommend eating *lots* of the following- the more good fats we eat and supply to our body, the quicker we might displace and replace the old, tired, free-radical containing ones. Many of us have been conditioned to be "fat phobic" and believe that all fats are bad for us. Nothing could be farther from the truth. These days many nutritionists are rethinking our dysfunctional relationship with fats. Yes, the bad ones are terrible and should be eliminated from our diets. But good fats are actually highly desirable and we should see them as our friends- not our enemies. This is a new view for many, but I think it is important that we stop thinking that all fats will make us fat. The evidence is overwhelming that it is not so! So what are some of these good fats?

Avocados are a rich source of vegetable fats that are unprocessed and undamaged- I think avocados are a great food, and I recommend eating lots of them! Fish oils of course are renowned for their healthy omega-3 fats. These can be extremely beneficial to your health, especially if your diet has been deficient in omega-3s, as so many are today. For vegetarian source omega-3s, fresh flax seed oil (available refrigerated in any health food store) is wonderful, and is an important nutrient-dense oil that is useful for homemade salad dressings or as an oil/fat "condiment" on steamed veggies, a baked potato, or anything else. Think of it as a healthy substitute for melted butter. Hemp seed oil is also a great vegetarian oil with many health benefits. I also really like coconut oil. Coconut oil hardens when kept below around 80 degrees, and has a butter like consistency. It is relatively stable to higher temperatures, so it can be used for sautéing or baking. Try it instead of margarine or butter if you bake muffins or banana bread, in your next pie crust, or in other baked goods. For heart healthy fats I am also a fan of unroasted almonds and other nuts and seeds. Almonds, pumpkin seeds, walnuts, and others can contribute healthy oils to the diet. Try and source the freshest nuts possible and keep them stored away from heat, light, and humidity to keep them as fresh as possible and to prevent rancidity from occurring.

Eating a nutrient-dense diet that has plenty of antioxidants, fresh healthful lipids, lots of pigments, and plenty of trace minerals and vitamins is a common sense and smart way to ensure healthier, productive mitochondria. This is really a key component to unlocking gummed up, less efficient energy production on the cellular level. Avoid refined sugars, fried foods, hormones, and artificial additives such as Aspartame and MSG and you will be doing your mitochondria- and your overall health- a huge favor!

Many nutritionists strongly feel that our food, and not supplements should be the foundation and mainstay of any program that aims to build, optimize, and sustain our health. I agree with this wholeheartedly. Yet for many, our metabolism has gone so far out of whack that sometimes more 'drastic' measures need to be taken. In order to 'jumpstart' a really stuck metabolism, sometimes additional nutrients- in other words, supplements- can be quite helpful for the short term till we get back on track. Once we are back on track, usually a really healthy diet will suffice to keep us there. So, if you are one of those people who could use some additional helping hands, here are some further recommendations and reminders as to what nutrients are most needed by our mitochondria.

Key Mitochondrial Nutrients for Energy Production

Omega 3 fatty acids (for mitochondrial membranes)
Lipoic acid (antioxidant membrane protection)
Co Q 10 (energy production)
L-Ribose (energy production)
Pyruvic acid (raw material for energy production)
Creatine (energy production)
Magnesium citrate (enzyme facilitator)
L- Carnitine (raw material transporter)
Vitamin E (antioxidant membrane protection)
Vitamin C (antioxidant)
B_1 (Thiamine), B_2, (Riboflavin), B_3 (Nicotinamide, Niacin) (energy production, co- enzymes)

Please notice, that at this point I am making a point of not giving dosage recommendations here. My feeling is that we are all so different in our lifestyles, genetic backgrounds, current health situations, medications we may be on, etc. that it would be irresponsible of me to try and give you dosage levels. Your best bet would be to go to your doctor or another health care provider who is knowledgeable about supplements, and most importantly, who knows your personal health and medical situation.

As you can see, there are a lot of options available to you in order to jump-start and tune up your mitochondrial environment. With the right help you can improve their functioning considerably, leading to more energy and in many cases to dramatic weight loss.

Part II

Cellular Dormancy

Metabolism Asleep at the Wheel

Chapter 5

Cellular Dormancy- An Introduction

The key to optimizing metabolic functioning is the process of rescuing or "waking up" tired cells from their state of struggle or slumber. I call this condition of depressed metabolic functioning, "cellular dormancy". Cellular dormancy simply refers to the condition where cells have gone from a normal level of metabolic functioning to a level characterized more by energy storage and conservation. Rather than actively expending energy in order to be ready to act and respond appropriately to external conditions and needs, such cells become our bodies' 'couch potatoes'. To some degree cellular dormancy is nearly universal in conditions of extreme weight gain, toxemias, altered thyroid functions, disrupted endocrine or hormonal states, and many other chronic disease states.

The causes and conditions that contribute to cellular dormancy are numerous. Some toxin exposures, especially to low levels over time, are well known to interfere with cellular respiration or energy production. In particular, heavy metals, such as lead, mercury, arsenic, aluminum, cadmium and others are well known to depress cellular energy production. So too does pesticide exposure. Another common cause of cellular dormancy is chronic under-hydration. Other causes include essential fatty acid deficiencies (EFAs are vital for healthy cell membranes and mitochondrial membranes.). Iron and other trace mineral deficiencies can also contribute or directly result in cellular dormancy. Additional adverse influences can include artificial hormones such as estrogens and progestins, other prescription drugs such as the "Statins" (widely prescribed to lower cholesterol levels), metabolic poisons such as fluoride (known to inactivate over 60 enzymes), chlorine, and carbon monoxide. A common nutritional cause has been trans-fats, prevalent for many decades in most fast food and junk foods in the form of partially hydrogenated oils such as margarines and shortenings.

The job of most cells is to perform specialized functions, such as secreting hormones or building proteins. In the case of muscle cells, it is to contract. In order to do these jobs, they all require energy, which is usually generated "on the spot" within the cell, in structures called mitochondria. It is here, in the mitochondria, where this crucial energy needs to be produced, that cells often face their biggest challenges and their "weakest links".

Cells that are struggling, dormant, or "asleep at the wheel" are like a fire that has been "damped down". With less available oxygen, the fire's intensity scales back and the burning slows down considerably. This is an apt analogy for a slowed down metabolic state. Another useful analogy taken from fires would be the type of wood that is being used for fuel. Country folk know there is a huge difference among different types of wood. "Hard woods" such as oak or ash or maple or locust- denser, harder woods- burn hotter and longer than "soft woods" such as pine or aspen. As we will see later, the more nutrient-dense foods help our metabolic fires burn hotter or more efficiently like harder, denser wood.

Fortunately, cellular dormancy can be overcome. Through a combination of nutrition, exercise, supplements, and lifestyle changes, stuck cells can be made to "get up off the couch" and begin to function again. When the metabolic brakes are removed, cells begin to wake up from their slumber, and they start to do what they are meant to do- burn calories more effectively, utilize oxygen and nutrients more efficiently, and act healthier in an overall way. When cells process nutrients and use oxygen to generate energy more efficiently the result is obvious: excess weight is shed effortlessly and the person has more abundant energy and vitality. What is the key to unlocking the puzzle of cellular dormancy? It is a nutrient-dense diet.

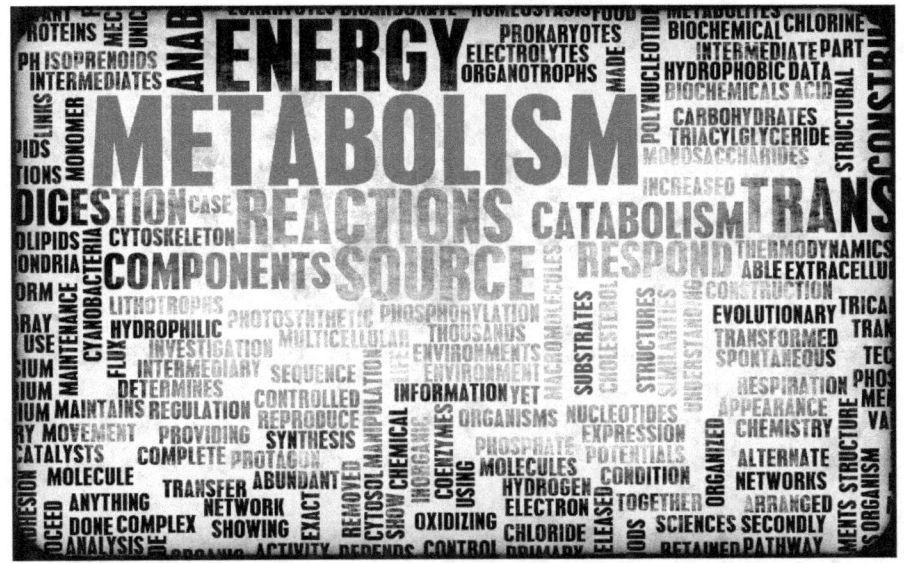

Chapter 6

Cellular Dormancy: Metabolism Asleep at the Wheel

For the vast majority of people, weight gain is due to one key factor- their cells are less efficient at producing energy. Instead of burning calories and releasing their energy as heat, many people's bodies switch to a "conservation" mode. In this state, people store their energy- as fat- instead of using it to fuel their metabolic needs.

When the metabolism is depressed, people tend to be sluggish, feel cold easily, have low energy, are poorly motivated, and often, are overweight. Frequently such people experience symptoms including depression, lack of confidence, apathy, or unnecessary fears. This state-which I call "cellular dormancy"- refers to tissues that are literally falling asleep, and can affect any and all organs of the body. It is for this reason that symptoms can vary considerably from person to person.

Why do some people's cells slow down and conserve calories instead of remaining more active? The answer may in part lie in their nutritional environment. In order to be healthy and active, cells need consistent "messages" that there is an abundance of available nutrients handy for them to do their work. At the same time, in the presence of toxins and other stressors, it is only natural that our cells may want to "go to sleep" rather than deal with a poisonous, toxic, or unsupportive environment. Drugs, including many prescription medications, food additives and chemicals, poor diets, hydrogenated oils, food allergies, hormonal imbalances, menopause, refined carbohydrates, ethanol, and chronic emotional stress can all contribute to a toxic cellular environment. Cellular dormancy is often the inevitable result.

Unfortunately, many people's diets today contain relatively high levels of substances that the body either does not need or want. And often their diets are low in key vital nutrients as well. This is one of the main problems with the SAD, or "Standard American Diet". Diets high in processed, chemical-laden foods are often deficient or marginal in nutrients needed to keep our metabolisms functioning in high gear. When our metabolism slows down, we burn fewer calories, and may shunt fats, carbohydrates, and even proteins into fat storage.

Cellular dormancy can be a quite complex process, and may vary from person to person- both in its causes and in its solutions. Nonetheless, there are several common principles that can dramatically help improve and "unlock" cellular dormancy resulting in weight loss and improved health and vitality. In the following chapters we will examine some of these principles and explain how you can put this understanding to work for you.

What Are The Risks From Cellular Dormancy?

A cell that is struggling to remain metabolically active and efficient in the face of nutrient deficiencies or other stresses is at risk for cellular dormancy or shut down. Another way to think of cellular dormancy is that the cell's metabolic activities are slowing down, or becoming less efficient. Sometimes I say that these cells are falling "asleep at the wheel". If a cell is not producing adequate energy in the form of ATP, it is not efficiently burning calories. In fact, cellular dormancy is another way of saying the person's metabolism has become sluggish. In many cases, weight gain is an obvious result: calories that are not being "burned" for energy are being stored as fat instead.

As we've discussed previously, the metabolic state of a cell is subject to many influences- both favorable and unfavorable. Some of these are environmental, meaning that they originate outside of the organism- some examples might include various chemicals, many prescription drugs poor nutrition, toxins, etc. Others originate *within* the organism itself- such as hormonal imbalances, autoimmune illnesses and other pathologies.

An energy deficit in terms of cellular energy production is clearly going to have an adverse impact on our overall health and sense of wellbeing. We constantly need to produce adequate or optimal amounts of energy to meet the myriad demands of the body. As we have discussed, cell reproduction, tissue regeneration and growth, hormone production, the beating of your heart, tissue repair and wound healing, and in fact all the physiological processes of your body require a constant input of energy, supplied in the form of ATP. When your ATP supply is inadequate to meet your body's needs, an energy deficit occurs. Chronic fatigue, lack of motivation, depression, fibromyalgia, and even heart disease and some cancers may be linked in part to a lack of cellular ATP and its consequences.

Cellular dormancy is an easy way to describe and understand what is going on with a cell that is not operating at peak levels. Essentially dormancy means asleep, or at rest; volcanoes that have not been active for long period of times are typically referred to as "dormant". However, it is understood by geologists that even a dormant volcano can sometimes come back to activity. So the good news is that even cells that are dormant are potentially able to bounce back and wake up as well. In fact, as we will be seeing, a "nutrient-dense" weight loss program can be specifically designed to help facilitate this bouncing back.

Scientists are well aware that there are numerous metabolic poisons present in our environment. Pesticides such as insecticides are a well studied group of chemical agents that do their lethal work as metabolic poisons by shutting down cellular respiration in insects and other pests. Some scientists believe that even trace levels, such as can be found in some foods, may have subtle, and possibly cumulative effects in humans on our metabolisms as well.

Other known or suspected metabolic "disruptors" include heavy metals (lead, mercury, arsenic, cadmium, aluminum, and others), plastics and many of the chemicals used in their manufacture, EMF radiation (such as from cell phones and home computers), PCBs, fluoride, chlorine, some prescription pharmaceutical drugs, "excitotoxins", such as Aspartame (NutraSweet™) and MSG, and hydrogenated oils (trans-fats). Workers in industries that are involved in the manufacture and production of some of these chemicals are potentially at risk, as well as many of us who buy and use them. As you can see, many of the most commonly used chemicals of modern life are potential metabolic disruptors, so that it is virtually impossible to completely avoid them.

Clearly there are innumerable opportunities and instances for toxic exposure available to all of us! Carbon monoxide, an odorless gas given off by incomplete combustion of fossil fuels- is a potent metabolic poison- and can be generated by a poorly ventilated fireplace, first or second hand cigarette smoke, or your old car's engine. Leaky stoves, furnaces, and car exhaust pipes can put you and your family at risk. Even breathing the fumes when you are pumping gasoline into your car can expose you to benzene, a fuel additive that is a known metabolic poison.

Many scientists and researchers are drawing the conclusion that at least some of the maladies of modern life may be related to this unprecedented chemical exposure. Some cancers, nervous system disorders, immunological problems, environmental sensitivities, and even obesity may have origins or close relationships with chronic or acute low grade chemical exposure. But the good news is that we can take many steps to minimize our exposure, neutralize the negative effects of some of these influences, and shore up our cellular defenses. In the following sections and chapters, you will learn specific strategies and dietary guidelines to help unlock cellular dormancy.

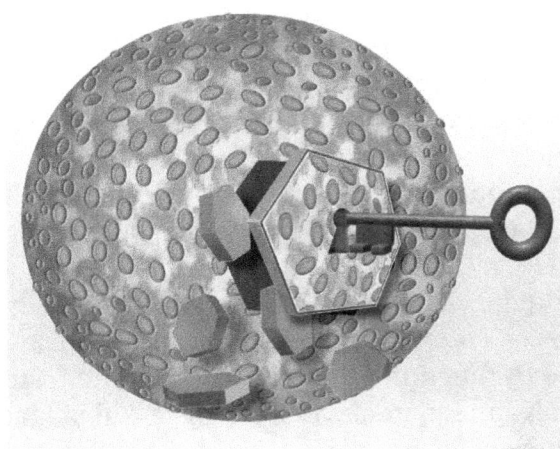

Unlocking Cellular Dormancy

The key to optimizing metabolic functioning is the process of waking up the tissues and organs from their state of slumber, a process I refer to as "unlocking cellular dormancy". While the causes of cellular dormancy are numerous, the solutions to unlocking cellular dormancy are also readily available. As we will see, a nutrient-dense diet is one of the most effective, common sense approaches we can take.

Clearly it is important and helpful to identify what is causing your cells to become dormant or sluggish. We have already listed several of the most commonly thought of potential causative agents such as certain heavy metals, some commonly encountered industrial chemicals, and even common at-home substances such as garden insecticides, as well as every day appliances and gadgets such as home computers and cell phones. Modern life is surrounding us with metabolic challenges!

One of the most common contributors of cellular dormancy is chronic under-hydration. Many of us simply don't drink water anymore- or nearly enough. For many, our water is usually mixed in   coffee, tea, juice, pop, or other beverages. Yet adequately hydrated cells are a must in order for them to perform their biochemical activities properly. Drinking enough pure water is a simple, but important and positive step that you can take to help support your cells' metabolic efforts. And, since added chlorine and fluorine are also metabolic inhibitors, it is recommended you drink artesian or spring water if possible.

Another frequent cause of cellular struggles are essential fatty acid deficiencies (remember, cell and mitochondrial membranes require these to function optimally). Since the SAD diet typically doesn't supply adequate levels of these substances, essential fatty acid deficiencies are considered by many researchers to be extremely common today. Since cellular respiration and metabolism depend upon healthily functioning membranes, eating the right fats and avoiding damaged or processed oils (such as hydrogenated oils and overcooked, "fried" oils) is an important step in improving metabolic functioning at the cellular level. We will discuss this in more detail in the chapter on nutrient-dense foods.

"Unlocking cellular dormancy" is obviously a priority if we want to regain our vitality, health, and zest for living. Fortunately cellular dormancy can be overcome. The good news is that there are many "keys" that can help unlock our stuck cellular doors. Through a combination of nutrition, exercise, supplements, and lifestyle changes, our stuck cells can be made to "get up off the couch" and begin to function again. When cells begin to wake up from their slumber, they start to do what they are meant to do-burn calories more effectively, utilize oxygen and nutrients more efficiently, and act healthier in an overall way. When cells process nutrients and use oxygen to generate energy the result is obvious: excess weight is shed effortlessly and the person has more abundant energy and vitality.

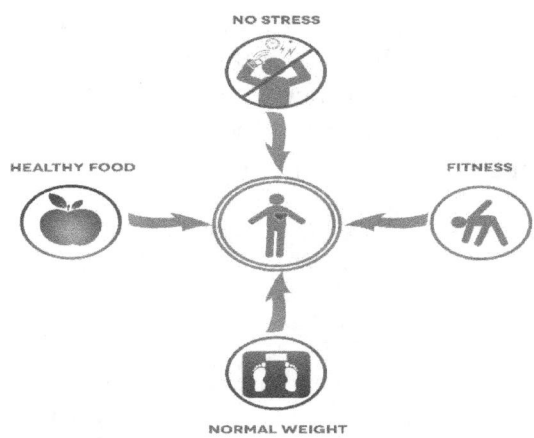

Chapter 7

The Therapeutic Spectrum

As I have alluded, there are a multitude of effective ways to address an inefficient, poorly functioning, or dormant metabolism. Some of these are what I call "common sense"- obvious solutions that we recognize as sensible and basic. Nonetheless, as I have written elsewhere, these days, common sense isn't all that common! Besides, even if we know something makes sense, we still can get so easily stuck in our habits that it often takes somebody stating the obvious to make an impact and get through to us.

In addition to some common sense answers to improving our metabolism, I hope to give you plenty of new ideas as well. This combination of obvious and new ideas constitutes what I call "the therapeutic spectrum". What this book is all about is providing you with a broad approach of effective strategies, behaviors, knowledge, and skills designed to create lasting lifestyle and metabolic changes.

The key to losing weight is to improve the overall metabolic efficiency of your cells so that they burn calories more effectively. The main approach is a combination of appropriate exercise and a properly healthy diet. Now let's take a look at the therapeutic spectrum in more depth.

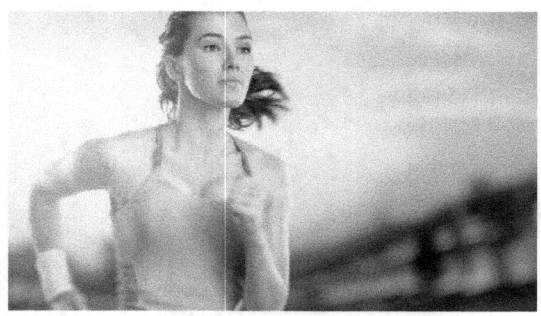

Exercise: Move It To Lose It!

Exercise! There is no doubt about it- exercise is absolutely essential for optimal metabolic support. Turning into a couch potato or sitting at a desk all day are simply not effective ways to stimulate your metabolism! The truth is, Americans get less exercise these days than at any time in history. Computers, televisions, and cars all mean we spend more time sitting and less time walking and moving. Why is movement important? Simply, we need to keep things circulating constantly; getting nutrients to where they need to be and getting wastes flushed out all require movement of the body. The flexing and movement of muscles squeeze and apply changing pressures on surrounding tissues. In addition, the exchange of key gases like oxygen and carbon dioxide require a constant flux of movement. Oxygen of course is necessary for aerobic respiration- the "breathing" that occurs within the cells, which is central to energy production. In fact, "cellular respiration" is simply another term for the transfer of electrons that occurs within the citric acid cycle- the key metabolic pathway within all cells. Getting oxygen in adequate amounts to all the tissues of the body is central to keeping your metabolism running and healthy.

Exercise helps improve the vital gas exchange within tissues so that our cells are "pumped" and flushed. Exercise also helps our circulation which improves the flow of oxygen via the hemoglobin in our red blood cells. It is also important for the movement and circulation of lymphatic fluid, which is an important part of our immune system.

Unlocking cellular dormancy means moving- consistently. Taking the stairs rather than the elevator, going for walks, riding your bicycle down to the corner store, doing yoga at home or in a class, swimming, dancing, working in the flower bed or garden- there are innumerable ways to keep yourself active. To paraphrase the well-known commercial: Just do them!

Moving more- in many people's cases, *much* more- is essential to any weight management program. A vitally important part of health is self-honesty If we can objectively look at how much we move our body, we might find there is a lot of room for improvement. We need to figure out ways to move more throughout our day- video studies of obese individuals show that they often become very good at conserving body movement. Such studies have shown that many obese people have developed "conservative movement strategies" and body postures that are excellent at conserving calories and energy expenditure. By moving minimally, the body's metabolism will likely power down as energy requirements are minimized. This is another way that cellular dormancy can come into play.

While a quick walk around your apartment or living room might be a wonderful thing for your metabolism for a few moments, it really takes more sustained movement to effect longer lasting or permanent metabolic changes or improvements. Many people do a quick couple of stretches in the morning- reaching overhead, bending deeply to touch the toes, that sort of thing- and again this is great. But compare that to following and keeping up with a teacher in a forty- five minute spin, Pilates, or yoga class and you can see there is really no comparison!

The point is, if you are someone who virtually never exercises or does much of anything truly demanding or "physical", then no weight program, eating plan, or diet will have as much of an effect on you. If you are physically unable to exercise at all, due to some physical problem such as arthritis or a bad knee or back, then I would say that focusing on making beneficial dietary and nutritional changes certainly does make the most sense. Then when you are able, begin to slowly, gently, and persistently make gradual progress with the help of a trainer, yoga teacher, or coach.

A nice thing about increasing one's physical activity level is that it doesn't have to be that dirty word, "exercise". Any enjoyable activity that involves repeated or sustained moving, walking, shaking, twisting, bending, or dancing will be helpful, and cumulatively so. The bottom line is that increasing your activity level can take innumerable forms and can and should be integrated into your life. Every bit helps!

So why do many people seem to resist exercise in any form? Interestingly, for many people there appears to be a vicious circle going on that keeps them from exercising or even moving more. It is not "normal" for the body to hurt. Yet for many people, this is their "normal". Many people have a greater or lesser degree of muscle achiness or soreness all the time that prevents them from becoming enthusiastic about exercise. Why is this? Surprisingly, the answer might lie in their mitochondria.

People with extreme cellular dormancy- those with really struggling or stuck metabolisms- actually use a different biochemical pathway within their mitochondria to produce energy. What happens is that they produce much of their energy via a less efficient method that ends up producing more of the metabolic byproduct called "lactic acid". And like most acids, lactic acid burns. This is the burn that athletes can feel after a particularly vigorous workout or for a normal person who pushes him or herself- we all know the feeling of having sore muscles after a day of skiing or hiking- especially if we are unaccustomed to such strenuousness. But for many people, there is a low to moderate background level of such soreness all the time as these folks just have higher levels of lactic acid present in their tissues. No wonder some of us have a real aversion to exercising!

Abnormal, persistent levels of lactic acid may be a real clue to weight gain in many obese people. Biochemists know that lactic acid is a byproduct of what is called "anaerobic" metabolism, which means the cells are not using oxygen as efficiently- often for a variety of reasons. Interestingly, many people with unexplained CFS (chronic fatigue syndrome) or fibromyalgia may have similar metabolic difficulties.

This is a vicious cycle at work. The increase in lactic acid may be from a metabolism that is doing more anaerobic work than normal. And this increase of lactic acid in turn makes it harder to be physically active, so the metabolism stays powered down, leading to even more anaerobic metabolism.

The answer to this vicious cycle is to employ the many nutritional and lifestyle suggestions that are in this book. Avoidance only perpetuates and prolongs the situation. Stretching, mild movement and exercise, lots of water, appropriate supplementation, and adopting a nutrient-dense diet coupled with abandoning once and for all the metabolic poisons and empty-calorie foods that are part of the SAD can all work synergistically to help turn around such a metabolic situation. The good news is that cellular dormancy can be overcome, and lactic acid levels can be reduced to normal levels with a return to normal cellular respiration.

Another important aspect of fitness is having decent muscle strength. So far what I have written about has been mostly about activity or movement- what we usually call aerobic activity. But fitness is not just about endurance; it is also about toning and strengthening muscles as well.

Actually using your muscles- whether digging a hole, pulling weeds, lifting a rock or a chair, doing a deep knee bend, or unscrewing a jar, is every bit as important as walking down the street. In fact, with respect to the topic of our metabolism and the subject of weight management, we could almost say "the muscles are more important than the lungs." This is true because muscle tissue burns many more calories than fat tissue does. In fact muscle tissue tends to have more mitochondria and produces more ATP than most other tissues.

One of the simplest things a person can do to help their metabolic cause is to pick up a couple of cans of food, or a pair of evenly matched rocks, or a couple of books, or a set of hand weights- and spend a few minutes each morning and evening lifting them and working out your arms and upper body. If you progressively challenge yourself and welcome "the burn" in your muscles then you will be positively impacting your metabolism immediately and profoundly without spending a cent.

Normally, we think about exercise as a way to "burn calories". But really, burning calories is only one benefit of exercise, and it is probably not even the most significant one. As we have discussed, exercise and movement do much more for us- such as improving tissue oxygenation and nutrient delivery by improving circulation.

Exercise has other important benefits as well. One is that it actually improves our sensitivity to insulin, so that our circulating insulin levels are lowered. This is really important and can help our metabolism greatly. Another benefit of exercise is that it lowers stress, and as an added benefit, can actually decrease stress-induced eating. Obviously this could be of great help in trying to lose weight!

Another important benefit of exercise is its ability to help with blood sugar levels. Exercise can also boost our metabolism in a general, overall way. This is a cumulative side effect of having improved circulation for delivering oxygen and other nutrients to our cells as well as carrying away wastes and toxic byproducts of metabolism. Finally, sustained exercise will actually increase the number of mitochondria within your cells!. This obviously has a big potential impact on the rate at which your body can burn calories.

My advice to you is, no matter how out of shape you are, start with where you are. Just because you haven't exercised in years doesn't mean you can't start- right now! It may seem hopeless, but the truth is, it isn't. Your cells-and your metabolism- will respond. The important things are (1) to begin, and (2) to continue. This is the main thing- to begin to be more consistent- and *persistent*. If you are like many overweight or obese people, you have probably become pretty consistent at things like "not exercising", or at consistently eating either the wrong kinds of food or too much of them. This book is about learning new, healthier habits and practices to be "consistent" at. And above all, it is my hope and wish for you that learning and incorporating such positive new habits will be an enjoyable and rewarding experience.

For a surprising number of people, making a change such as adopting an exercise routine or simply working into one's life a higher level of activity is just as hard, if not harder, than making dietary changes- and we all know how hard that is! People who already do exercise regularly probably can't understand why it is so hard for some to adopt a more active lifestyle, just like a lot of health nuts probably can't fathom why everyone doesn't eat like they do. The good news is that it doesn't matter what anyone else thinks! This is about you, and you are the only person you really need to satisfy! So, remember, the point of embarking on a journey of improving your metabolism isn't to feel guilty or to feel guilt-tripped or to feel judged or compared to others. What it is about is making changes, but only in accordance with your personal comfort levels. Whether we are talking about diet or your activity level, one should never feel pressure- only encouragement and support and hopefully inspiration and a confident belief in oneself.

Becoming more active will hopefully not feel like a chore or burden- just like adopting new, healthier eating habits should not feel like deprivation or punishment! **The hardest part of any self-improvement program is overcoming one's personal initial inertia**. This is why I emphasize taking small, manageable steps in the beginning. If we don't approach it this way, the whole undertaking may feel way too daunting, in which case we are likely to either not start at all- or, if we do, we may find ways to undermine or sabotage our sincerest efforts. Old habits are hard to break-which is why they are called, "habits". So, it is important to be gentle with ourselves, to set firm but realistic (and modest) goals, and to understand what I call "the psychology of our resistance".

Hydration

Drink plenty of water! Though this might sound like the kind of advice your mother might give you, there is also a sound scientific basis for this recommendation. Water is so important to our metabolism that I am giving it its own little section. Water provides the hydration and proper 'environment' necessary for optimal biochemical functioning. Being adequately hydrated is considered by exercise physiologists and other health professionals to be a critical component of any sound health regime.

The truth is, many Americans simply do not drink nearly enough water today. Soda, coffee, and other beverages are not a substitute for pure, "naked" water. Further, on a nutrient-dense program, it is considered more beneficial to drink spring water with naturally occurring dissolved minerals over municipal tap water that probably contains chlorine, fluoride, and other chemical residues. Chlorinated and fluoridated water is thought by some health professionals to be another metabolic straw on the camel's proverbial back. The truth is, chlorine and fluoride are both known to be metabolic poisons, so why ingest them if it is avoidable? Chlorine is never listed on a label of water or any other beverage and neither are the amounts, so why take a chance? And the same goes for fluoride as well. Pure spring or "artesian" water should not have either of these elements artificially added to it.

And if you want to be really serious about your health, many nutrition experts recommend bottled water from glass over plastic. We are starting to learn a lot about the additives in plastic containers, which can leach into our drinking water. Some of these so-called "plasticizers" are thought to be potent hormone disrupters. Water is an important starting point for being more proactive about your health. It is a great example of a simple, incredibly practical, and commonly overlooked aspect of our lifestyle.

Positive Thinking

Positive thinking! As I have discussed at length in the above section on exercise, there is often a psychological threshold that we may need to cross if we are to successfully undertake any kind of self-improvement program. Knowing our inner struggles, habits, patterns, resistance, and expectations is important if we are to successfully negotiate a new territory of change- whether it be dietary change, a new exercise program, or what have you. Many of us have gotten quite used to ourselves- even if we are not entirely happy with where we are at. Familiarity is comfortable; and this is something human nature seems to crave almost more than anything else. The unknown- even if it is for some form of "betterment"- can be really scary, and threatening to the status quo. As a result, many of us have become quite adept at "self- sabotage". We may genuinely want to drop that excess weight (or whatever our goal is), but when it comes down to making actual changes- and sticking with them- we may find that we come face to face with some interesting inner demons and their negative talk.

65

Who are these demons anyway? Often they masquerade as voices or messages of self-doubt, telling us that there is no point to trying, that we will fail anyway, that the effort and time are not worth it- that sort of thing. Usually they raise their voices when we are on the verge of succeeding- they begin clamoring when their old way of existing is threatened by new behaviors. Therefore, we could say that as we begin to reach our potential, the resistance from our past increases. Knowing that this is how self- sabotage often works can help us in our determination to stick with our goals.

It would seem that one of the best ways to plan for success is to anticipate it. In other words, most of us need to set really strong intentions if we are to meet our goals and overcome our resistance, complacency, laziness, or self-doubt about our capabilities. This is where positive thinking comes in! If we doubt we are capable, then we likely will find ways to prove that that assessment of our ability is correct. In this way, failure becomes a way of confirming that we were "right" about ourselves. If we "fail" to achieve our goals or to stick with our program, then this "failure" allows us to justify not having to give up our comfortable patterns and face the uncertainty of change.

Another way to look at this is that it is our nature to become comfortable or complacent with ourselves. Change is threatening because it means we will have to deal with a potentially "new" us, or at least, another, unfamiliar aspect of ourselves. For many of us, newness is more frightening than it is exciting. It presents us with challenges, new problems, and the hurdle of getting to know more about ourselves. All of these new situations require work, or effort. We often love the familiar because it keeps us from having to put energy into learning new things!

For all these reasons, we should respect the fact that changing our habits is not an easy task, and should not be taken lightly. Many if not most of us have had the experience of making a new year's resolution and not following through, quite possibly because our "resolution" was fairly frivolous and not taken so seriously by us. It is my hope that your resolution about obtaining genuine greatly improved health and weight reduction (if that is your goal) is something that you feel strongly about this time. In my experience, for many people it takes a bit of what I call "fierce determination"- a *really strong* resolution- to effect truly effective, lasting change.

This is the "positive thinking" that I mentioned at the beginning of this section. Success will ultimately depend upon your mindset- your true intentions. It is normal and to be expected that you will face moments of doubt, of re-considering your decision and of course, facing many inevitable temptations to either quit or cheat on your program. How you face each one and how you set your boundaries and how you keep on going will be the critical factors determining whether ultimately you continue improving your metabolic condition or if you abandon it and remain in a locked down mode.

Really there are only two crucial factors determining whether you stay with the program or not: (1) the strength of your determination at the beginning- in other words, how "badly" you want the results you will get if you work the program, and (2) how well you deal with the challenges and temptations you will face as you travel the journey. If you think about these things now, before you actually start making changes, you will very likely have an easier, more rewarding, and hopefully, more fun time on the program.

Part III

The Nutrient-Dense Diet

Eating As If Your Metabolism Mattered!

Chapter 8

What is Nutrient-Density And Why Does It Matter?

The Nutrient-Smart weight management system is based upon a very simple premise: if you eat optimally, you will start to optimize your metabolism, your health, your weight and your life. This is not a far-fetched or outrageous idea; rather, it is common sense wisdom that many have forgotten.

The most basic concept in nutrition is the old adage: "you are what you eat." This simple saying reflects the fact that every cell in our body- and virtually every atom and molecule- are ultimately derived from the nutrients we ingest. At its most basic level, we could say that if we are what we eat, then if we eat mostly junk foods, we will likely end up with a junky body. By the same token, if we eat truly healthy, optimally nutritious foods, we should end up with a relatively healthy body. Of course there are many other factors at work in our lives, such as genetics and lifestyle, but basically, this is a valid and sound approach to eating.

What is Nutrient-Density?

Nutrient-density refers to the nutritional "denseness", or concentration of nutrients in any given food. Foods that are nutrient-dense for certain nutrients deliver relatively abundant amounts of that nutrient of nutrients. This is analogous to a computer or chip with more "bytes" of information packed into it. These are foods that nutritionists commonly think of as healthy, beneficial, and useful. Nutrient- density offers us a useful guideline for determining which foods are optimally nutritious and hence, health-enhancing.

A nutrient-dense diet is essentially the exact opposite of the SAD, or Standard American Diet. The SAD is full of lots of "empty calories", meaning calories that are delivered without much in the way of accompanying nutrients. Sugar, and most other refined carbohydrates like white flour and white rice, as well as alcohol are classic examples of empty calorie foods.

But not just refined carbs contribute "empty" calories. Refined, or highly processed fats and oils are also culprits, similarly giving us calories, but little else in the way of necessary nutrients such as minerals and vitamins. By contrast, healthy fats can supply us with important essential fatty acids, which are essential for our health and well-being.

Why Does Nutrient-Density Matter?

Nutrient-dense carbohydrates, proteins, and fats are how we can get vital nutrients along with the calories we need. Our metabolism, as well as the various cellular structures, tissues, and organs of our bodies depend upon such nutrients.

But nutrient-dense eating is not just important because of the nutrients it supplies. Equally important are the molecules that a nutrient-dense diet does *not* supply. While our bodies *require* nutrients such as vitamins, minerals, essential fatty acids, amino acids and more, what we *do not* need should be examined as well. Our bodies have *no* need for molecules of aspartame, artificial colors, monosodium glutamate, synthetic hormones, fluoride, and countless others.

In the past it has been easy to dismiss most of these chemicals as unimportant but neutral or benign additions to our food supply. Certainly the food industry has spent considerable money and effort in trying to convince us that such additives are completely neutral and harmless. However, it might also be true that many such molecules could have actual detrimental effects on our metabolism and other cellular processes- especially when we consider their long term, cumulative and synergistic effects.

In this way, our nutritional needs should be looked at from two directions: how to get *more* of what we require for optimal health, and how to get *less* of what might be detrimental. And this is exactly what an optimally nutrient-dense diet will do for you. Naturally the food industries that profit from selling their additives and foods will vociferously disagree with this assessment.

Of course the final decision of what to purchase and what to put into your body is yours alone. This is a personal and private decision, and should be made based upon your own understanding of how your body works as well as your own intuition or insight of what is best for you. Unfortunately, there are many factors and pressures at work that make it challenging to sometimes live up to your beliefs and decisions- from clever psychological marketing campaigns designed to get you to buy certain products to the "peer pressure" of well-meaning relatives and friends. Ultimately though, the decision is up to you each time you reach for something to eat. This book is designed to help inform and support you in your quest for better health and quality of life.

You can probably already see that the principles of nutrient-dense eating are pretty simple. Calories actually require certain nutrients in order to be properly and efficiently metabolized. It is an established fact that most Americans are actually marginal or deficient in at least several essential nutrients including key vitamins and minerals. Nutrient-dense foods help to correct these deficiencies because they are generally the most excellent sources of specific nutrients; in fact this is actually the definition of nutrient-dense foods. Many of the commonly eaten foods from the Standard American Diet, by contrast, are nutrient-poor, leading to a situation where nutrient deficiencies can occur. **If certain nutrients are not available in adequate amounts, calories may not be metabolized as efficiently.** This of course, is the basic premise of this entire book.

It makes sense that nutrient deficiencies can lead to what I call "cellular dormancy" and consequent weight gain. Instead of struggling to make use of the little nutrient support available, the deficient individual's cells, tissues, and even organs go into "conservation mode". By slowing down and doing less work, these tissues will require less of the all too rare nutrient helpers. This slowing down and moving into conservation mode is precisely what I call "cellular dormancy". You can think of it as a powered down metabolic state.

Nutrient-Dense Principles

Nutrient-density is easy to understand and easy to implement. Instead of nutrient-poor, empty calories, most of your food's calories should be accompanied by naturally present, essential nutrients. Our food is where we should obtain most if not all of our vitamins, minerals, essential fatty acids, amino acids, and other vital nutrient needs. Yet sadly, most Americans are deficient or marginal for many of these. By contrast, a nutrient-dense diet provides optimal or high concentrations of these nutrients.

The principles of nutrient-density are simple. Eat mainly foods that are basically unprocessed and mostly straight from nature, with a minimum of tinkering. This means fresh non-GMO fruits and vegetables, whole grains, nuts and seeds, and if you like, organically and humanely raised animal products (meat, seafood, dairy). As much as possible try to avoid foods that have been highly refined as well as those that contain a lot of additives such as artificial flavors, colors and preservatives. Seek out the most nutritious foods and prepare them simply so that they will retain most of their natural goodness.

Once learned nutrient-dense shopping, cooking and eating is the easiest and most natural way to nourish ourselves. It is also the most satisfying and empowering way to eat because we begin to regain control over our bodies and our food choices. Modern food producers and vendors have learned to maximize their profits by cutting corners. Their food may taste good, but generally they rely upon chemical tricks- artificial colors, tastes, texture enhancers, preservatives, artificial or "natural" added flavors, etc. to make their wares last a long time and to look and taste appealing.

Unfortunately, processing in this way can compromise nutritional quality. By the time such food reaches your mouth, many of the vitamins, minerals, and other nutrients are frequently destroyed, lost, or damaged. At the same time, many of the chemicals used- preservatives, artificial flavors and colors, antibiotics, hormones, herbicides, insecticides and others- even in very small amounts- can damage or impair mitochondrial functioning and other delicate cellular processes. This can eventually have a profound effect upon overall metabolic functioning and efficiency. Years of eating a diet based on nutritionally compromised foods can lead to the consequences we see all around us- a country literally filled with overweight people, too many prescription drugs, and numerous other signs of poor health.

Putting Nutrient-Density into Action

Once you have made the decision to put more nutrient-density into your life, the actual implementation is surprisingly easy.
The beginning of your journey starts by clearing out the biggest metabolic obstacles and hurdles. After that, everything else is relatively easy.

What are the biggest obstacles, and why tackle them first? For an analogy, take the example of creating a garden from scratch. In order to grow a garden, you have to first clear an area, turn over the ground, pull out the weeds, etc. Only after the beds have been well prepared can we plant our seeds or put in our "starts". But before we can do any of the above, we must first clear the area. This means if there are any large rocks, pieces of wood, old tires, or other debris blocking or choking the site, we must remove them in order to get to the ground below. In the same way, if you are going to make any future headway with your metabolism, first you should get rid of whatever is "keeping your brakes on".

What are the biggest metabolic brakes facing Americans today? Actually there are numerous metabolic "poisons" or toxins known to impact metabolic functioning. But to prioritize and simplify things I think the four most prevalent and preventable that so many of us face today are (in no particular order): **(1) synthetic hormones (2) refined carbohydrates- both table sugar and fructose (3) hydrogenated and highly processed oils and (4) Aspartame (aka, NutraSweet).** If you can eliminate these four nearly ubiquitous metabolic poisons from your diet, you are a long way towards "taking off the metabolic brakes". From here, you can begin to enjoy the ride to better health and weight normalization that will result from unlocking your state of cellular dormancy.

Whether you can eliminate these four substances from your diet is of course, up to you. Many people have learned to keep these metabolic toxins out of their diets and have no problem doing so. The catch is, all four of these poisons are extremely common in the standard American diet. Therefore, in order to successfully lose weight in the Nutrient-Smart Weight Management Program, you have to be motivated enough to take the responsibility and time to read labels. In other words, you have to be willing to do without many of the brands and foods that you have come to love or depend on.

I do not pretend that this easy for everyone. To be perfectly honest, it likely means a fairly radical overhaul of your present diet. The good news however, is that you do not have to have a "perfect" diet overnight. This is exactly why *The Nutrient-Dense Eating Plan* is divided into tiers of increasing denseness. In fact, *I encourage you to go at your own pace.* If you honor your own comfort level with the changes, you will increase your odds of success tremendously. Later I will offer further strategies and more specific methods for overcoming the tendency many of us have to "self-sabotage" our good intentions and sincere efforts to make positive, lasting changes in our lives.

Increasing the Denseness of Your Diet with Exceptional Foods

After "clearing the debris" from your body (by eliminating hydrogenated and processed oils, Aspartame, refined carbohydrates and hormones), you can begin to add in nutrient-dense foods little by little. This will ensure that your cells are getting quality nutrients and adequate *quantities* of nutrients. Many of the most nutrient-dense foods are really "super nutrient-charged foods". I call these foods "exceptional" foods, and they are the heart of *The Nutrient-Dense Eating Plan.* They are also the heart of the *Nutrient-Smart Weight Management Program* as they can literally wake up your body, and help transform your cells from a state of cellular dormancy to one of efficient and optimal functioning.

Learning to incorporate nutrient-dense, "superstar" foods can be fun and rewarding, but initially, maybe a bit daunting for some. We are all different in how readily we embrace new, untried things. Some of us are a bit more adventurous or open minded, whereas others may be a bit more conservative and cautious. There is really no "right or wrong" when it comes to trying new things or adopting a new style of eating. We need to respect who and where we are at- and we should each go at the pace that is most comfortable for us. This is precisely why *The Nutrient-Dense Eating Plan* is designed in tiers or steps; and we are encouraged to take them at whatever speed we feel is right for us.

With that in mind, I would like to now introduce you to a few of the nutrient-dense "superstars" that are available. Later in the book we will discuss some of these in more detail, especially the ones that have particularly important roles to play in supplying specific metabolism- supporting nutrients. However, we don't really need to look too deeply at specifics at this point. Increasing the overall consistency and quality of the diet is the main point: the more dramatic the change, the more profound and obvious will be the impact on your metabolism.

A Nutrient-Dense Superstar Checklist:

Vegetables: Almost all vegetables are moderately to highly nutrient-dense- especially when organic and raw or lightly cooked

Fruits: blueberries, raspberries, (all berries, really), apples, bananas, citrus, kiwi, mango, pomegranates, organic pineapple...basically all fruits, esp. when organic

Oils: coconut oil, flax seed oil, cod liver oil, wheat germ oil, hemp oil, organic grass-fed butter, extra virgin olive oil

Carbohydrates: blackstrap molasses, brown rice, millet, quinoa, organic baked or boiled (not fried!) potatoes (when the skin is left on), yams, raw honey

Proteins: (note: all animal products must be organic to eliminate hormones, antibiotics, and other metabolic toxins) Eggs, elk, lamb, buffalo, wild caught seafood (not farmed), some sushi, any organic meats, liver, unpasteurized cheeses and yogurt, almonds, sunflower seeds, walnuts, pine nuts, sesame seeds, peanuts, tempeh, beans, lentils, peas, brown rice, millet, quinoa.

Miscellaneous: nutritional yeast, sea weeds, miso, bee pollen, spirulina, chlorella, nuts and nut butters, many spices and herbs, teas, sprouted grains and seeds, dark chocolate (small amounts).

and antibiotics. Organic poultry is likewise difficult to find (especially in most restaurants) but health food stores and many farmers markets do carry it.

As you can see, nutrient-dense eating may necessitate some rather major shifts in how you approach food, meals, shopping, cooking, and dining out. Yet, with a little planning, practice, and patience, nutrient-dense eating is every bit as easy as your old, more familiar way of eating. The truth is, a little effort and sacrifice is necessary in order to gain the huge benefits of improved health and the body you want. If you are clear about your goals, and you have the genuine desire to reach them, then nutrient-dense eating will answer your wishes. It can also open you up to an exciting and rewarding new world of eating. And, in the process, it can empower you to have a healthier new appreciation and relationship with food.

Nutrient-dense eating is really the cornerstone of the *Nutrient-Smart Weight Management Program*. Our diets are really the most important factor influencing our metabolism because it is what we do every day that has the single biggest cumulative impact upon us. When we eat, what we ingest sends messages-both obvious and subtle- throughout our body, to each and every cell. Our food conveys messages of quality, caring, and intention. Our food choices also tells our body whether our intention is to nourish and uplift it through high quality food- or it can convey a message that our body is an appropriate and proper receptacle for "junk food"! This is exactly why earlier I spoke of "self-esteem" and "dignity" as vitally important concepts in nutrition and health. The signals we get from our food choices says a lot about whether or not we are walking our talk or not with respect to how we really see ourselves. Getting NuDe is about coming into alignment with our expectations about ourselves and what we deserve.

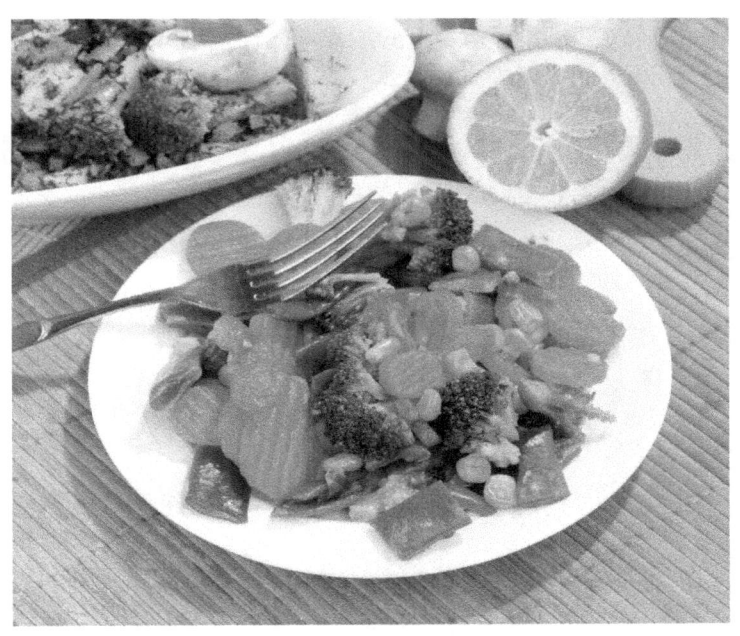

Chapter 9

Eating for Weight Management

What sets this program apart from any other is its emphasis on quality, nutrient-dense foods to nourish and support our metabolic machinery. We have already discussed the other principle aspects of the program- exercise, drinking plenty of water, and the right mental outlook. Here I will discuss and outline in more detail some of the specific foods and nutrients which can support optimal metabolic functioning. Please remember- this is the heart of the program!

Improving the overall metabolic status of your body is the real goal of eating super healthily. A nutrient-dense diet will ensure that your body remains well-nourished while your body's metabolism is supported so that it comes back up to speed quickly and safely. If you follow this eating plan, I promise you will be pleased with the results.

A Word about Supplements

In addition to a nutrient-dense *diet* I will also be recommending certain specific nutrients or supplements as an addition to the foods you eat. While it would be ideal if food alone was sufficient to kick a sluggish metabolism back into high gear, some people's metabolism either has been dormant for so long or is in such a deep state of slumber that it may initially need an extra helping hand- a sort of nutritional jump-start. The nutrients I will be recommending are all widely considered extremely safe when used in the amounts given. However, as we will talk about further, it is always smart to consult with your physician and approach taking any supplements with a bit of intelligent caution. Carefully nudging your metabolism into wakefulness is what we are after here; this should not be a heavy-handed or stress-provoking approach. Rather, working with your metabolic state should be done gently, mindfully, and with respect for the uniqueness of your body.

One key thing to keep in mind is that we are all slightly different- biochemically, genetically, and metabolically. Therefore, even though the supplements that are recommended are generally quite safe and have a remarkable track record, there is always going to be the occasional, rare, exceptional person who could have an idiosyncratic reaction. Again, this is why a doctor's approval and even on-going supervision is a good idea- especially if you are taking any prescription medications. As always, the information in this book is not intended to replace your doctor's advice. If in doubt, do not take any supplements without getting medical approval first.

But, before we get to the supplements, lets zero in on the main part of the program for unlocking cellular dormancy- eating a nutrient-dense diet.

Your Nutrient-Dense Weight Loss Program Options

In this book we have briefly looked at human metabolism- what it is, how it works, and what can affect it- for both better and worse. We have also examined cellular dormancy- the situation where our cells' metabolism starts to "power down". As energy production struggles to keep up with the normal demands of life the metabolism slows down with the somewhat predictable result of weight gain and often other accompanying health issues. In particular we have discussed some of the causes and ways to address this pervasive problem. We have also discussed nutrient-density- and have seen that eating with our nutrient needs in mind can present a commonsense approach to eating that holds real promise for addressing and even reversing cellular dormancy. So what is next and how do we put nutrient-dense eating into practice?

I believe there is a spectrum, range, or continuum of options available to the serious person who wishes to proactively take their health up to the next level (or levels). Some of us are more comfortable going in small, easy-to-manage steps. This incremental approach can be much less daunting and threatening than an "all at once" leap. But then again there are others who may be ready to "give it all they've got" and "go for it" in a fairly aggressive way. This kind of decision is of course very personal and individual and many factors can weigh in on which style is best for you. A well-considered and informed decision should take into account many factors, but in the end, I think your health and safety should always be the bottom line. Therefore this might be a decision best made with the help or assistance of your physician or other trusted and knowledgeable resources. In the end, it is your body and your decision, but please think it through carefully!

This type of consideration is true of both drastic dietary changes as well as adding new supplements or even a new exercise program to your health regimen. Our bodies are often in a fairly delicate state of balance- even when they are out of balance! So making a change that can potentially shift things–even for the better- can sometimes have stressful or unintended consequences for us. For this reason, it is always a good idea to be carefully monitored and supervised.

In this book I designed several "tiers" or stages that describe how to transition to a more and more nutrient-dense lifestyle. At each stage we become progressively more careful and attentive to our food selections and eating choices.

So, with that in mind, what I would like to do here is outline four different scenarios for addressing cellular dormancy. If your body is out of balance and in need of either a tune up or a jump-start then there are several ways you can go about it. Since there is a continuum or a spectrum of options, please take my scenarios and suggestions with some latitude. The point here is that these phases are just a few recommendations to give you some ideas as to how to get started. This is not a program that is "etched in stone" and you are strongly encouraged to modify and make changes to suit your needs, lifestyle, and personal preferences. Now, let's take a look.

PHASE 1
Lose the junk!

The first level, or tier really focuses on just eliminating most of the basic "junk" and bad stuff. This reflects the analogy I used earlier about clearing the debris out of our future garden plot. Instead of old tires, stumps, and big rocks, I am referring to the metabolic debris that is so common in most people's diets these days- the hydrogenated oils, refined carbohydrates, artificial sweeteners like NutraSweet, fried fats, and the synthetic hormones typically found in all commercial pork, dairy, beef, and poultry products. I would also include artificial colors and GMO ingredients in this category. When these are eliminated- usually by making some very basic initial changes and by switching to organic animal products- then these first steps have been taken. This is a great start and really needs to be adopted by everyone on this program- but there is still much more to be done in order to become strongly nutrient-dense.

PHASE 2
Creative Substitution Time!

In the next tier we actively start to bring in more nutrient-dense choices. I call this process "creative substitution" and it really helps with the overall quality or nutritional denseness of the diet. What we are doing here is taking our diet to the next level by finding better quality foods to replace some of our current "normal" ones. The point of this phase or stage is that we are not really changing "how" we eat very much- we are essentially eating the same way- we are simply "upping the ante" by finding more nutritious versions of our standard fares.

Examples might be substituting almond butter or organic peanut butter for commercial peanut butter made with sugar and hydrogenated oils. Other examples could be substituting coconut milk or almond milk for commercial, hormone laden cows milk, or even making your own almond milk from soaked almonds in your blender. Another example might be using sprouted grain breads which are much more nutrient-dense than ordinary white flour breads. Or try brown rice or quinoa in place of white flour pasta or macaroni. Another example of creative substitution would be using coconut oil in place of margarine or butter. There are countless such examples of ways to substitute healthier food choices to increase the denseness of your eating options.

PHASE 3
Bring on the Super Foods!

Finally, as our diet really begins to become even more nutritious, we start to actively add in nutrient-dense "super foods". This is where our diet really starts to take off and becomes much more nutritionally dense. This is also where things can start to get really interesting! If you are an adventurous type of person and quite open-minded when it comes to eating and trying new things, then you will probably embrace this phase with gusto. However, if you are a much more conservative and "food cautious" person, then quite frankly, this is where I could lose you!

Some examples (see appendix: "Super Foods") here might include adding spirulina or chlorella to your smoothies, and using items such as nutritional yeast, sea weeds, bee pollen and flax oil as condiments or "add-ins" to your meals to really boost your nutritional intake. Fresh juices (from your juicer, not from the store), sprouts, and raw goat's milk are other examples of foods that might become incorporated as part of your normal diet at this level of commitment. You might also more actively seek out some of the more nutritious vegetables for your meals-such as beets (greens as well as bottoms), kale, and the cruciferous vegetables such as broccoli and Brussels sprouts.

As you can see, not everyone will be ready (and many will never be!) for this kind of dietary lifestyle. For others it is a matter of taking it slow and making changes gradually and comfortably. Whatever you choose, the only thing that really matters is going at the pace that is most suitable and comfortable for you. There is no "one size fits all" here!

PHASE 4
The Raw/Live Food Diet

For those who are highly motivated and ready, probably the fastest way to lose weight (provided you are healthy enough to handle it and have checked with your health care provider) is to adopt a mostly raw or "live" food diet. In my experience, the quickest way to jump-start a sluggish or stuck metabolism is to go 80% or more raw. This means eating a diet that is predominantly composed of lots of fresh fruit, lots of salads (using "live" flax oil), plenty of vegetables, avocados, and fresh juices (yes, you will need to borrow or invest in a juicer). You can also eat plenty of raw (unroasted) nuts like almonds and walnuts and seeds such as sunflower seeds or pine nuts.

Although it might appear quite extreme, in this approach virtually everything that is eaten is largely unprocessed, simple, clean (meaning, chemical-free), unheated (uncooked) and nutritious. With a diet like this, and with plenty of fresh water being drunk and some exercise incorporated- and perhaps some additional supplemental support in really stubborn cases-I can almost guarantee you will see pretty dramatic results in a very short time! This is especially true if your diet up to now has been like most people- meaning virtually everything consumed is cooked or processed. When you really think about it, most people these days eat a very small percentage of their diet in the raw or "live" form.

Now I want to acknowledge that the raw dietary approach is pretty extreme. I am not denying that. Let me be blunt: this is probably not the best approach for most people! This is not because it isn't safe or effective, because it is. Rather, it is just too darn "extreme" and hard to stick with for most of us- especially considering the day- to-day realities of the "social" aspects of eating. Having said that, the live food diet does represent a viable and real option that is available for motivated people who can fit it into their lifestyle.

I feel it is very important to present this as an option and as something to consider. Remember- even though this approach represents an extreme dietary style, it is very effective and when supervised properly, quite safe. As I said, it represents an extremely effective way to drop weight quickly and safely. In one fell swoop you cut out most of the biggest metabolic challenges: no gluten, no dairy, no refined carbohydrates, and no hormones.

Adopting a live food diet doesn't have to be a long- term commitment either. If your metabolism is severely out of whack and you would like to give it a good jump-start, even an "experiment" of a few weeks duration is likely to get you on track so you start dropping weight fast. If you can last a couple of weeks I'll bet you will start to feel so much better and so much more energetic that you will have little trouble going further.

Remember, how you go about this is totally up to you. While there are many strong advocates out there of eating 100% raw, that might – or might not- be what is best for you. For some, 100% is actually easiest because then there is no chance of "slipping"- the boundaries are clearly drawn and there is a clean sense of what is and what isn't allowed.

For others, especially when you are new to this, it might be more appropriate to strive for 75% to 80% raw rather than fully 100%. If this is the case, you might be more comfortable experimenting with the right mix of mostly raw, live foods and a smaller amount of other, cooked foods such as lentils and brown rice and a few other things to help your body "adjust" and transition. Again, there is no "one way" for everyone and what is most important is to trust and respect your body and lifestyle. As I've said before, it would probably be wise at this point to have some supervision and guidance, especially if you have any health issues or are on medications.

Some of the mainstream dietary programs and many "experts" will likely frown on such an approach. Amongst dieticians, nutritionists and others it is inevitable that some will say such an approach is potentially dangerous. One objection might be that it lacks enough protein, for example, to be healthy. Others might raise the concern that the recommendation of eating lots of fresh fruit could supply too much sugar and could be detrimental to one's health. So, let's discuss these concerns.

First, and most importantly, virtually all studies done on the metabolic "dangers" of fructose used pure crystalline fructose- isolated and purified- or as high fructose corn syrup. This is an unfair comparison as isolated fructose is worlds apart from eating fresh fruit! We should remember that with fruit nature supplies us with fructose along with plenty of fiber, minerals and vitamins, enzymes, and other nutrients. Let's be clear: eating fresh fruit is not even remotely the same as eating isolated or purified fructose!! Besides, the amount of fructose in fruit is small compared to the purified stuff that is in, say, a typical soda. You would have to eat 3 apples, 90 cherries, 5 bananas, or 9 cups of strawberries to get as much fructose as in one 20oz soda. And again, with the fruit you have much slower absorption due to all the fiber and enzymes.

As for protein, a raw diet can supply enough for almost all normal people- and if you really need extra, you can simply modify your diet. If you feel you need extra protein, you can get plenty from additional eggs, some cooked brown rice with beans, etc. Don't forget that nuts and seeds are also good protein sources.

Many nutritionists feel that most Americans actually eat way too much protein anyway, which can be hard on the kidneys, liver, etc. Besides, going raw for just a few weeks to jump-start your metabolism should not be a problem at all for the vast majority of people. Throughout history countless people have fasted or gone on very low protein diets for similar, limited periods of time with little or no long term problems. Vegetarians and vegans seldom in actuality experience protein deficiencies, and in fact are typically much healthier than their meat eating counterparts, especially considering the higher risks for such diverse conditions as gout, arthritis, cardiovascular disease, obesity, many cancers, kidney problems and other conditions that can be associated with high animal protein diets.

In conclusion, countless people have shown that a raw or living food diet is not only safe, but a healthy way to improve or "tone up" your metabolism, especially as a "jump starting" technique. Whether you adopt this style or not to eating is up to you. What I would say though, is that no matter what, anytime you can eat something fresh and raw- whether it is a handful of cherries, a fresh peach or a pear or an apple or banana, or a super salad- you will be doing your body- and your metabolism- a big favor!

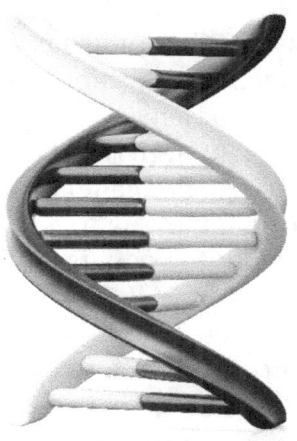

Chapter 10

Food As Information

There is a famous saying that is supposed to go back at least as far as the early Greek Physicians, who were famous in their day as the most progressive thinkers of their time regarding medicine and healing. They said "Let food be your medicine, and let your medicine come from your food." Today we can apply this same thinking. In unlocking the puzzle of weight and metabolism today, food still holds all the cards.

Letting food be your medicine and knowing that you are what you ingest are old, wise, tried and true statements. Interestingly, they are now supported by ultra-modern scientific research and understandings of how our genes work.

Our genes are the "information bits" that are coded within large DNA molecules, which are in turn incorporated within twenty three pairs of chromosomes that are found in almost every one of the cells in your body. Our inherited genes constitute what is called our unique "genome". These genes handle our physical acutely sensitive to any number of drugs, alcohol, etc. There are many such examples, such as to what extent our nervous system might be sensitive to MSG or aspartame (NutraSweet), or gluten, or a host of other potential irritants. How we respond to environmental or nutritional challenges are things that can change- for the better or for the worse during our lives. This is great news- that we can put to good use!

What is exciting and relevant to our conversation about metabolism and weight is this relatively recent understanding that food actually "talks" to our genes. What we now know is that food not only acts as a conveyor of nutrients- it also acts as a conveyor of information. Food contains bits or "bytes" of information that it constantly communicates to the genes in our cells' nuclei. In this way food has a very direct influence on our cellular environment.

This makes a lot of sense if you think about it. Food is evolutionarily an extension of our environment and reflects back to us information about the seasons, the quality of the soil, and much more. The quality as well as the quantity and availability of different foods communicate an incredible amount of information to our cells, all the time. Our environments can be relatively clean or relatively polluted-and they can be relatively chemical-free and nutrient-rich, or relatively gummed up with metabolic toxins, wastes, and chemical compounds of all kinds. Even nutrient-deprivation from lots of empty-calorie foods sends a message. And now we know that our cells "understand" these seasonal and environmental messages and respond accordingly.

This is a real breakthrough in our understanding of nutrition. First we learned that food carries calories- units of energy. Later we discovered that food supplies us with vitamins- organic molecules that our bodies cannot produce themselves and which need to be supplied from our diets to ensure good health and even to keep us alive. In addition we learned a lot about the structure, roles and functions of minerals, proteins, fatty acids, and other important molecules. Finally we discovered the roles of antioxidants, pigments, fiber, enzymes and other nutrients in keeping us healthy.

Therefore, this latest discovery represents a shift of thinking and a real expansion of our understanding of just how nutrition works. Instead of just being the carrier of physical elements of nourishment, food is also a carrier of information as well!

Today, the messages that food is capable of conveying to us are more starkly divided than ever before. For example, our food can signal to us very positive messages. One message could be of nutritional abundance, of strong membranes and the abundance of plenty of energy-making molecules (substrates, in chemical terminology), of anti-inflammatory phytonutrients (like turmeric), and of antioxidants. That is one clear, consistent message that our cells- and our metabolism- loves to hear. A message of abundance and of a plentiful and reliable supply of nutrients will likely result in healthy cells, tissues, and organs that are more "relaxed" and "confident". The result is a situation where we are ready to function in a state of relatively good overall health and wellbeing. Less hardship and deprivation and therefore less stress communicates to our body that it does not need to worry, or to store lots of fat for lean times. Our hormonal levels actually change and respond to reflect a state of nutritional abundance and less nutritional "stress".

On the other hand, our food choices can also signal something entirely different and communicate an altogether different message to our body. Such a message could be something like: "hey, nutrients are scarce, so we need to conserve them and slow things down a bit, but in the meantime, there are plenty of breads and pastries available and other foods that have plenty of calories, and here are a bunch of meats and dairy products – so we won't starve, and so what if there are a lot of hormones along for the ride? And for good measure we also have a lot of really

95

tasty fried foods- who cares if the oil in them is old and oxidized? Artificial flavors and colors? We'd better just accept them as part of the package. Beggars can't be choosers, so let's eat as much as we can of these empty foods, and if hard times come, at least we'll have plenty of body fat to live off for a while."

It's really pretty simple. Here we have two vastly different approaches to supplying our body with the food and fuels it needs, and two vastly different messages being conveyed to our body. Every day our genes literally receive hundreds of these different and contradictory communiqués from our world of gardens, fast food restaurants, junk food brands, health food stores, organic markets, convenience stores, farmer's markets, etc. and have to make sense of all this inputted information. Our weight, our metabolism, and our health all depend upon the signals- and mixed messages- our bodies receive and how our body interprets them and ultimately reacts to them.

We are what we eat. Depending upon the messages, calories, toxins and nutrients (or lack of) that we ingest, our bodies respond either with energy, vitality, creativity, and inspiration, or with a sense of heaviness, lethargy, and lack of drive. In other words, our bodies operate somewhere along a continuum within the bookends of an optimally functioning metabolism on the one end and a defeated, struggling, dormant metabolism on the other. This is the playing field that our body occupies. We can learn and choose to eat in a way that supports our health and energy, or we can eat in the SAD (Standard American Diet) fashion and risk being part of the 67 % of Americans considered medically overweight or obese.

In terms of our diets, most of us aren't perfectly good, and most of us aren't perfectly bad either. But wherever we find ourselves, there is probably room for improvement, especially as far as our food habits go. The point of a metabolic approach to weight management is simply to show you exactly how easy it is to make more consistent choices in your diet so as to nudge your metabolism in the right direction by giving it the right information, nutrition, and messages. Eating much more consistently in a nutrient-dense manner is the single most important thing most of us can do to incorporate the principles of "let food be your medicine" and "you are what you eat".

Waking up from cellular dormancy is within reach for everyone! Eating more and more nutrient-densely and transitioning to a nutrient-dense eating lifestyle can make profound and lasting changes in one's metabolism- and waistline. Taking the clamps off of a dormant metabolism by eliminating synthetic sex hormones alone can help a lot, as one example. Another example could be eliminating dairy or gluten from our diet- if we are genetically sensitive to these food groups. The truth is, many of us are and don't know it. In reality you won't know, either, unless you try. You might be quite surprised what kinds of results these kinds of shifts can make. As the saying goes, "the proof is in the pudding."

This kind of diet directly reflects our old adage "you are what you eat". Eating almost exclusively live foods sends a message to your cells and genes via the enzymes and pigments that freshness is going to be "the new normal". Live foods cause the body to "liven up" and wake up from their slumber. Because this style of eating focuses on fresh, live, enzyme-rich "raw" foods, there is simply far less room for highly processed and ubiquitous "dead" SAD foods including white flour baked products such as breads, pizza, bagels, muffins, cookies, cakes, pasta, etc. Similarly there is no longer "room" for empty-calorie products made with refined sugar such as candy, desserts, soda, ice cream and the like. Such a diet sends a clear and focused message to your body and targets your cells for their "metabolic make-over".

In my experience, many people have a deep resistance against making radical changes to their diets. Many folks are deeply suspicious of the suggestion that they may need to give up their favorite comfort foods and happy meals. Many of us are deeply attached and possibly even addicted to many of the basic brands in our diets. In fact, many people strongly resist changing what or how they eat even if it is literally killing them.

Even if we are used to eating such processed foods for many years, our bodies never really quite "get used to them". Instead our genes and our metabolism make adjustments to accommodate this style of eating, making compromises that lessen our health, and in general trying to make the most of a difficult situation.

This is a shame, because many of the foods that we love to eat are highly processed, artificially flavored, textured, preserved and synthetically colored "fake foods" that are not even remotely natural and certainly not necessary for our health or life. It is an ironic but economic reality, that 'real" foods, such as fresh vegetables and fruits, almost always lack the marketing dollars and hype that characterizes many of the trademarked brands that seduce us as consumers with glitzy advertising and big budgets.

Most of us are not aware of the depth to which we crave or depend upon certain foods. Food companies have gone to great lengths over the past several decades to identify molecules that literally have addictive properties when we ingest them. One of the best known is the "flavor molecule", monosodium glutamate, or MSG as it is more commonly known. MSG tricks flavor receptors into thinking food tastes are "brighter" and more exciting than they really are, so food manufacturers who use less expensive and often over-cooked foods love it. As far as "information" goes, these are messages that are repeatedly telling us lies and falsehoods!

MSG is the #1 most commonly used food additive in the world precisely because it artificially amplifies or exaggerates taste perception. For this reason it is called an "excitotoxin" because it excites or stimulates certain nerve endings and receptors. Unfortunately there is also a toxic side to this substance, as it can literally over-stimulate nerve cells to exhaustion or death in some cases. Ironically virtually all processed foods today use MSG, and many researchers feel there is a definite link between obesity, overeating, altered taste perceptions, and MSG use.

Commercial salad dressings, soups, ketchup, sauces, condiments, prepared meats - virtually anything you can think of has it added in these days. And virtually everything on the menu at any of the big fast food restaurant chains contains it. Even so called "happy meals" use MSG in their food, condiments, "secret sauces" etc. Children- and their vulnerable, developing nervous systems- often get way more than their fair share of this excitotoxin as food companies vie for their lifelong brand loyalty and future dollars. Unfortunately there are no laws to require label disclosure of this additive-which literally adds insult to injury! So even if you are a dedicated label reader you will usually not know if it is in a product or not!

MSG is just one single example of thousands of food additives-most of which have never been tested for safety or potential health effects. What we should remember is that most such food additives are chemicals- molecules that our bodies do not need and do not 'recognize' as anything natural and which are seldom or rarely encountered in the natural world. By ingesting them in our diet, aren't we giving an entirely new and unprecedented message to our genes? If 'we are what we eat', then do we run the risk of becoming more 'artificial' and less natural ourselves?

Are we telling our genes that we are ok with cutting ourselves off from the natural world of our ancestors and that substituting fake tastes, synthetic foods and ingredients is ok? What about the artificial hormones- synthetic estrogens that we eat on a regular basis with our pizza, hamburgers, and chicken? What kind of messages does ingesting these chemicals on a regular basis say to young boys' and girls' bodies? And what about the building blocks and key nutrients our bodies need? Are we running a risk of diluting these vital nutrients by eating loads of empty calories? What kind of messages are we giving to our bodies? Is this what we want to communicate to our genes?

These are important questions and ones that are well worth contemplating. It is up to each one of us to choose for ourselves what kinds of fuel and nutrition and messages we decide to put into our bodies. Most of us never stop and ask these sorts of questions- we are too busy with our lives, making other kinds of decisions, and putting out fires of all sorts in our busy lives. So we just eat what is convenient and cheap. But it might be worth remembering that taking care of our bodies is still a responsibility that we each have within our reach, and that we can make fresh, informed decisions at any moment that could have big consequences and implications for our health and quality of life.

Smoking is a great example. For many decades, Americans smoked cigarettes quite unaware of the profound health risks they posed. Eventually, when enough evidence had come out, many people realized that this seemingly pleasurable habit was really causing a lot of misery and simply wasn't worth the risk. Today we might be at a similar juncture with respect to our growing awareness of the risks of eating too many empty calories, too many synthetic hormones, too many pesticide residues, too many artificial sweeteners, too many artificial flavors, and too many artificial dyes, etc.

Food is something we do every day. Every cell in our body depends upon our daily food choices to provide them with the raw materials they need to do their jobs. Food is many things- a source of pleasure, a way to nourish ourselves, a socially important ritual, a part of our identity. But it is also the source of a steady stream of messages and information that we send to every cell in our body- about how we think, what we value, and how we intend to treat our most precious possession- our body.

Whether we do this with thoughtful awareness and intention or unintentionally is up to us. Ignorance might be bliss- or it might be a path to obesity, diabetes, and poor health. Let's turn our attention now to some of the different foods that we have access to every day, and how they can affect our metabolism- for better and worse.

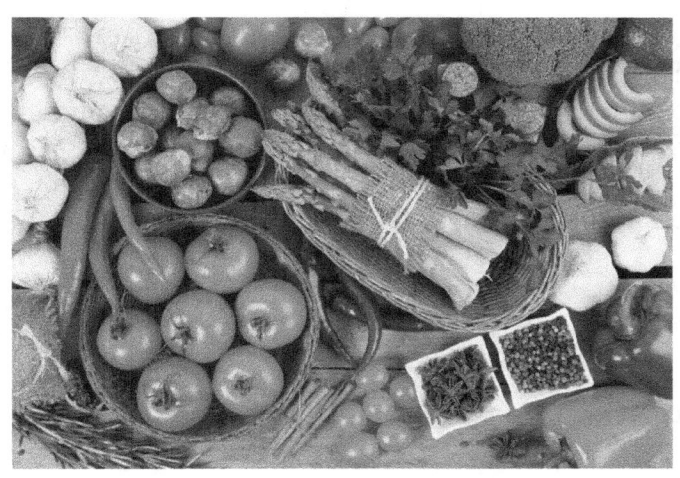

Chapter 11

Optimal Eating:
How *Nutrient-Dense Eating* Can Maximize Your Metabolic Success

I discussed earlier what the basic principles of nutrient-density are and why it matters so much to our metabolic goals. Here I would like to spell out more clearly the parameters of what optimal nutrient-dense eating looks like in "real life".

Please keep in mind that our principle health goals are to (1) lighten any toxicity or metabolic load on the mitochondria on the one hand, and (2) ensure that most if not all of the nutrients required throughout the steps along the energy producing metabolic bio- pathways are provided in optimal amounts. I feel that both of these goals are easily attained if one has an optimally nutrient-dense diet. Now let's take a look at what such a way of eating might actually look like.

The best way to look at nutrient-dense eating is to always seek out nutritional *quality*. If you consistently identify and consume the most nutrient-dense carbohydrates, proteins, and lipids (fats and oils), as well as the highest quality "superfoods", you cannot go wrong. We will identify and discuss many of these foods in more detail shortly.

The Metabolic No-Nos

First, however, let's start with a short but solid handful of no-nos. I would like to get these out of the way so we can move on to the more positive, "fun" stuff- the good foods! Eliminating non-nutrient-dense foods and metabolically inhibiting junk foods and empty-calorie foods are very important first steps. Cutting the bad stuff out of our diets is vitally important for "taking the clamps off" a stuck metabolism and clears the way for progress to occur. This is the analogy we mentioned earlier as if we were going to create a beautiful garden full of lush healthy vegetables or flowers. In order to start a garden, we must begin by clearing away the debris that might be choking the site. So before we can even plant our garden or till the ground, we first need to remove any old stumps, big rocks, or old tires or paint cans that might be on the site. Once the site is cleared of debris, then we can actually dig the beds and prepare the soil properly.

So, what are the metabolic "debris" foods that we need to clear away and get out of our bodies? The good news is there really aren't that many- in fact as we shall soon see, the number of good, metabolically supportive foods far exceeds the categories of "bad" foods.

First, because of important concerns surrounding hormones in food, absolutely no non-organic dairy is allowed at all. This is also true of any chicken product, including eggs. And guess what? This goes for beef and pork as well. In fact, essentially *all animals* raised and sold these days by the commercial dairy, beef, pork, and poultry industries are subjected to inhumane factory farming methods, which routinely use large quantities of growth hormones- typically synthetic estrogens. Agri-business also uses extreme amounts of antibiotics to ward off disease- not to selectively and carefully treat individually sick animals but in an indiscriminate shotgun effort to minimize diseases. Many of these chemicals can act as metabolic poisons- and therefore indirectly contribute or even directly cause cellular dormancy to occur. Simply put, eating non-organic meat, poultry, and dairy makes shedding unwanted weight much harder. Therefore such foods are not allowed in this program- pure and simple. To put it bluntly, these foods- and the hormones they contain- along with our addiction to refined carbohydrates- are likely *the* major culprits in our country's runaway obesity epidemic.

If you think about it, this makes perfect sense. The food industry uses these hormones to fatten and mature their animals quicker, so they can "turn them over" faster and make a quicker profit. Make no mistake about it- these hormones are potent chemicals, and many are well known to induce cancers and other tumors in addition to fattening up industrially raised animals. A lot of evidence suggests that today's problem with obesity is due in large part (no pun intended!) to our ingesting these hormones on a daily basis with our milk, cheese, eggs, bacon, chicken and hamburgers. By eliminating all such hormone-containing foods (however, you can substitute certified organically raised meats and dairy) you will be taking a huge step towards unlocking your dormant metabolism.

Pretty much that is it for forbidden foods. Oh, fried foods are virtually 100% out. They are a metabolic nightmare as we learned in the section on oils. And, if you really are serious, most breads and baked products should be eliminated too. There are a few notable exceptions of acceptable breads, so all is not lost. I will recommend some of the most nutrient-dense breads in the appendix. There really are some, truly nutrient-dense breads- you just have to know what they are! But otherwise you will need to strictly curtail almost all baked products for now.

On this eating plan I also strongly recommend that you avoid NutraSweet^{tm} in any form. That means: no sugarless gum, and no diet drinks at all- especially if they contain Aspartame.. NutraSweet^{tm} might sound like a good thing- after all it is in so many so called "diet" foods and drinks and has the healthy sounding "nutra" in its name. And it saves calories, right? Well, sorry, a lot of evidence strongly indicates that Aspartame may not be a benign (harmless) additive, despite what the food industry would desperately like you to believe. According to many clinicians it acts as an "excitotoxin" and can cause all sorts of problems with our nervous systems, with our digestion, and with our metabolisms. If you consume it now, I hope you will stop. It is also addictive for some people, so if you love it, you might find it hard to give it up- which certainly might be a sign that you have an addiction to it. If you want to continue to use Aspartame-containing products, of course that is your right, but if you want to strictly follow this program and really lose weight, I strongly urge you to "cold turkey" it and give the stuff up. It really has no place in your nutrient-dense eating program and is likely counterproductive to your weight loss and health goals.

I'm sorry to have to be so blunt, but let's face it, SAD food as usual probably hasn't cut it for most of us up to now, or you wouldn't be reading these words. I'm not saying you can *never* eat these "forbidden" foods; in fact once you reach your goal you can certainly relax your guard a bit if you want. But if you really intend to follow this plan and if you are really, truly committed and determined to lose weight safely, healthily, and efficiently, then my suggestion and recommendation is that you 'just say no' to the above food categories for a few months. Try it and see what happens- you might just be astonished at how much better you look and feel!

Let's be completely honest here. This is the hardest part of any diet- giving up familiar, tasty, easy-to-find foods that have always been part of your life. I know this can be challenging. I know this can be daunting. And I know this can feel depressing-

for a while. But if you can get over the initial phase, you will be just fine!

Most of us are "highly social creatures". We hang out and work and socialize with friends, loved ones, family members, co-workers, fellow church goers and others who may not understand or sympathize with what you are trying to do. It is virtually certain that they will be eating and serving and offering most if not all of what you are trying so hard to avoid. Let's face it- this can be awkward, and this can be hard. No one likes to feel "rejected"- even if it is for positive, healthful reasons- and no one likes to be the one to do the rejecting either!

Sometimes those around us can even feel threatened or insecure when confronted with a friend or loved one who is doing something "different". They might take your dietary changes as a rejection of who they are and what they believe and value. And you might occasionally find yourself in the uncomfortable position of having to defend yourself or justify your new food choices. This is to be expected; don't think that everyone around you will be happy and jumping for joy for you as you try to improve your health. This is why I always stress that mental preparation is really crucial for this – or any- weight loss plan. Expect to face some challenges and you will have a much better time of it.

Who are the ones who most succeed at programs that require change? **The people who succeed are usually the ones who are prepared to weather the storms of criticism, ridicule, sabotage, and lack of support**. Often people who are sincerely trying to lose weight are shocked to find that their so-called friends actually will try to undermine their efforts. No one wants to be left behind. Getting healthy and committing to one's one welfare can be an interesting journey! You might even learn a few new things about your friends and social circles!

Let's complete this part of the no-no foods section with a brief summary and reminder. As you will see in a few moments, the great foods that are allowed and encouraged are much more numerous, diverse and fun than the "bad guys". But bear with me- it is really important to clearly state what not to eat as much as what to eat. So many people have asked me for years "what can I eat?" and "what should l avoid?" So to avoid this kind of confusion, I am spelling it out for you. All I ask is that you give this a sincere try for a month or two - cut out what I am recommending you cut out and eat what I am recommending you eat- and see for yourself if your metabolism doesn't do a 180. I'm willing to bet you will be amazed- and delighted.

The Worst Foods for Your Metabolism:

- Alcohol
- Aspartame (NutraSweet^{tm)}
- Bad oils: commercial cooking oils that are non-refrigerated, including corn oil, soybean oil, canola oil, peanut oil, and cottonseed oil.
- Fried foods (chips, fries, chicken...)
- GMO corn, soy, sugar (these are the biggest but there are many others)
- High Fructose Corn Syrup
- Hormone-containing animal products (i.e. any non-organic: eggs, chicken, milk, cheese, pork, beef)
- Monosodium Glutamate (MSG)
- Partially-Hydrogenated oils, fats, shortenings and margarines
- White flour (and virtually all baked goods)
- White sugar

Your Metabolically-Friendly Foods

Now for the fun part! As you'll see, there are a great many wonderful, delicious, and interesting metabolically-friendly options available to you. You'll quickly see that the best part of eating "nutrient-densely" is that whole worlds of eating pleasure and adventure await you. It's understandable that people might anticipate and worry that a "diet" is about deprivation. The interesting irony is that when you eat a nutrient-dense diet you actually eat so much better than before- simply because nutrient-dense foods are pure, simple, and of the highest quality and nutritional value. In fact, as noted, we don't even count calories on this program, because nutrient-dense calories are not the real problem or issue- only empty calories are! This is the key- finding the best quality, healthiest and most nutritious carbohydrates, proteins, and fats. If you follow this simple rule, you cannot go wrong!

I would start by saying that every day I would strive to eat a minimum of several servings of fresh fruits and/or vegetables- and really more if you like; in fact, whatever is fresh, tasty, and appealing should be incorporated and enjoyed. I recommend snacking on fresh fruit whenever the mood hits you- from a nutrient-dense point of view, you can have virtually unlimited access! Focusing on the many kinds of berries and the juiciest types of fruits- from kiwis to all kinds of citrus to pineapples to mangoes, to peaches and plums and berries to melons and cantaloupe- it's pretty hard to go wrong eating as much of these as you want. Eat them alone as a snack or incorporate them into healthful smoothies or juices.

The abundant amounts of fiber, enzymes, minerals, vitamins, and bright, colorful antioxidant pigments present in fresh fruit "trumps" any concerns about the naturally occurring sugars present and renders these concerns as inconsequential. Think of the tradeoff: after all, you are giving up cookies, candy, cakes, ice cream, and sugary beverages for fresh fruit. I think it is very hard to find fault with wholesome fresh fruit! There is really just no comparison. The same goes for vegetables- eating a wide variety of all types in salads is a smart nutrient-dense eating strategy and should be a frequent and enjoyable component of your diet.

In terms of dressings for salads and vegetables, I usually use fresh flax oil or a very fresh, cold- pressed flax blend as a base, and often mix it with some high quality extra virgin olive oil. I highly recommend incorporating fresh oils such as flax seed oil generously, as they will nourish your cellular and mitochondrial membranes and help a wide variety of tissues. This is definitely a case of "the right fat does *not* make you fat". If you have "fat-phobia", please don't let it extend to the healthy oils-or avocados! They are your very good friends, not your foes! Just remember the huge difference between these excellent cold pressed oils and the other highly processed no-no oils!

If you are a meat eater, then there are a large variety of nutrient-dense options available to you. Many wild, cold water fish such as salmon, cod, and sardines are great. Try and stay away from farmed fish, mercury-containing types and endangered species. Lamb, buffalo, and elk would be my main meats of choice. In particular the liver is very nutrient-dense- ask your butcher for buffalo liver- it's loaded with B_{12}, iron, and other nutrients. He may have to special order it for you, but it is worth it!

Organic eggs are also welcomed – and are recommended quite highly in *The Nutrient-Smart Program.* Boiling or poaching are the healthiest ways to cook them! If you have access to free-range eggs from a neighbor or farmer's market, go for it! And please note- eggs that are certified "organic" does not mean they are necessarily truly free-range. They are a definite step up from ordinary eggs, but "organic" chickens may still be kept under quite crowded and stressed conditions.

I personally also recommend raw milk- particularly goat's milk, as well as any cheese, yogurt, or butter that might be made from it. You will probably not find these in stores, but if you look for them you might find a neighbor, local farmer or farmer's market with these. If these are handled with care and kept clean, they should be safe and highly nutritious. These are all very nutrient-dense foods and I recommend them highly- *if* you eat dairy and *if* you are not dairy sensitive. In their "raw" forms such foods can be very metabolically supportive, unlike their commercial, pasteurized and homogenized counterparts.

I also heartily recommend you eat plenty of nuts and seeds. Raw, unroasted sunflower seeds and almonds are both extremely nutrient-dense foods, and so are pine nuts, walnuts, sesame seeds, pumpkin seeds, pistachios and others. Nut butters made from these are great too. Freshly made almond milk is a wonderful treat too, and can be used in cereals, as a beverage, or as a base for a nutrient-dense smoothie. For a non-dairy milk or creamer, try coconut milk- it is wonderfully creamy and can be used in lots of creative ways as a milk or cream substitute.

All spices and condiments and especially many herbs are nutrient-dense for a wide variety of antioxidants and other phytonutrients. Herb teas are also encouraged, especially as they can contribute further molecular diversity into our diets. Green teas in general and matcha in particular are reputed to have thermogenic (heat, or metabolism generating) properties. Ginger and garlic and turmeric root are greatly renowned for their culinary and healing qualities. Cinnamon aids insulin's effectiveness, and so is especially desirable for many with blood sugar issues.

I am an especially big fan of seaweeds- particularly varieties such as dulse, kelp, hijiki, arame, wakame and others. These can often be purchased in larger pieces for use in stir-fries and soups, and are also available powdered and packaged for use just like you would salt and pepper. Later I will show you some of the many ways you can incorporate these "super foods" into your meals to make them more exotic and nutritious.

Especially in the fall and winter months, brown rice, quinoa, and millet comprise three of the main grains that can be used as inexpensive gluten-free staples of a nutrient-dense diet. I frequently use them as a meal base to which I add my favorite nutrient-dense condiments such as flax oil, nutritional yeast, sea weeds (often dulse or kelp flakes or powder), and many times, salsa or hot sauce.

Served with millet or brown rice, a hearty stir fry-using coconut oil and with plenty of lightly sautéed vegetables, onions, organic mushrooms, and garlic and/or ginger- makes a consistently delicious and superbly healthy meal throughout many a winter night with nearly infinite combinations and variations. You can even throw in a handful of almonds or other nuts for added texture, crunch, and added protein and nutritional value. These types of easy "skillet dishes" are equally delicious as either vegetarian/vegan or with a little meat or fish added in. I sometimes also add some tofu or tempeh (a soybean product) as inexpensive meat substitutes. You can find recipes and suggestions for these kinds of dishes in *The Nutrient-Smart Weight Loss Program.*

There are also many different kinds of nutrient-dense specialty foods- foods that are uniquely nutrient-dense for one nutrient or another. Often these lend themselves for use as supercharged condiments. One example is bee pollen which is full of trace nutrients from flower pollen. I frequently use a spoonful as an "add-in" or supplement to smoothies- but you can also put it in oatmeal or organic unsweetened yogurt or applesauce. It is also easily mixed or added to nut butters and spreads. Other foods in this category include chlorella or spirulina (powdered blue-green algae superfoods with unique nutritional and anti-inflammatory properties), and nutritional yeast- a fantastic source of many B vitamins and several key minerals with a unique nutty/cheesy taste.

I am putting fresh ("live") juices into a special class of their own, though they can also be thought of as concentrated fruits and vegetables. I am a huge advocate of juicing, and encourage all of my seriously nutrient-dense friends to try and get in a rhythm of juicing at a minimum of 4-5 times a week. If you are genuinely desirous to gain energy and lose weight, fresh juice, such as a carrot/veggie blend or a fruit juice or fruit/veg blend every day will really help "wake up" your dormant cells. Fresh juices are super concentrated sources of pigments such as chlorophyll and others, and contain loads of minerals, vitamin C, healthful sugars, and especially live enzymes- important molecules that catalyze chemical reactions in our bodies. In the "you are what you eat" paradigm we could say that a breakfast consisting of fresh juices is a case of liquid live juices acting like an alarm clock- entering your body and waking up your sleeping cells!

I think you can see by now that this is not a diet about deprivation at all. There is a lot of room for gourmet dining. Even some sushi is welcomed as a nutrient-dense food category. And, yes- as far as sweets go, dark chocolate is definitely...on the menu! Unless you live somewhere where there is virtually no access to healthy food, going Nude or NuDe (nutrient-dense) is relatively easy. The transition, which might feel a bit daunting at first, is really easy once you take the first few steps. It may surprise you how easy and yes- enjoyable- it is to get Nude! Instead of feeling deprived, I bet you will feel empowered and delighted with how enjoyable, delicious, and rewarding eating all this wonderful food can be. And feeling better, getting healthier and losing weight will be the best of bonuses!

Greatest Foods for Your Metabolism!

- Apples
- Beans, legumes, lentils
- Bee Pollen
- Berries- fresh or frozen
- Brown rice
- Buffalo meat, liver
- Cayenne powder
- Coconut oil
- Coconut milk
- Coconut water
- Eggs (must be organic and free range)
- Flax oil
- Fresh fruits (apples, berries, kiwis, melons, mango, pineapple, etc)
- Fresh Goat's milk
- Fresh Greens (lettuces, baby spinach, arugula, kale, etc)
- Fresh Juice (carrot, veggie blends, fruit blends, wheatgrass)
- Fresh Veggies
- Garlic
- Ginger root
- Green tea

- Jalapenos and other hot peppers
- Kombucha
- Lemons
- Millet
- Nutritional Yeast
- Nuts, seeds (preferably raw, unroasted), nut butters
- Onions (yellow and red)
- Quinoa
- Radishes
- Salsa (fresh)
- Sauerkraut (fresh, "live")
- Seaweeds (e.g. kelp, dulse, many others)
- Shiitake mushrooms
- Spirulina (and Chlorella)
- Sprouts (alfalfa, broccoli, mung, radish, sunflower
- Squash (winter and summer)
- Umeboshi Plum vinegar
- Wild Oceanic fish
- Yogurt (unsweetened, made from raw milk)
- Honorable mention: (small quantities) dark chocolate, red wine, microbrew beer

See, I told you there would be a lot more great metabolic foods compared to the terrible ones! Now I know many of you are wondering what the heck you will do with some of these foods and ingredients. Later I will give you some ideas of how to incorporate some of these ingredients in delicious, nutrient-dense recipes that will also nourish you and support a more active, "awake" metabolism. You can also learn more ways to incorporate these super foods in *The Nutrient-Dense Eating Plan*.

I hope that you are getting a good idea by now at just how this program works. **By eliminating the "bad" foods and actively pursuing the "good" ones, I think that you can see that it is possible to dramatically turn around your internal cellular environment- and your overall health**. For many of you this kind of change of eating might feel quite drastic- but I sincerely hope that you might be starting to look at this with a sense of curiosity, adventure, and even excitement. Changing how you eat can be quite an adventure, and I encourage you to approach this journey with a sense of optimism and open mindedness. You are worth it! All it really takes is a bit of courage, an open mind, and the belief that you deserve it. If you really want to lose weight, then changing how and what you eat could be the most powerful, helpful, and important step that you will ever take. It has the power to change your life- for the better- forever!

Chapter 12

Some Nutrient-Dense Eating Suggestions

Most "diet" books have extensive recipe sections. In fact for many it is a good way to "pad" a sparse book and add pages. This book will be a little different. I will certainly give you some meal suggestions and recipes, but more than that I hope to give you the confidence and inspiration to create your own recipes and meals using high quality, nutrient-dense ingredients.

Building Confidence: Learning to Trust Your-self in the Kitchen

What will be obvious to you as you look these recipes over is that most of these are not true "recipes" in the traditional sense of the word. Instead what you will find here are examples that you can use as jumping off points to create your own meals. For example, you will see that there are usually no exact measurements. There is an important reason for this. One of the messages I am trying to convey is the importance of developing a confident, healthy relationship with food. This means learning to trust yourself- and the food ingredients! My recipes are really more like suggestions to point you in the right general direction. As a teacher, I feel the highest goal is to help people learn from their own involvement and trust their own experience. We often learn best from our mistakes! Everything you try doesn't necessarily have to turn out perfectly the first time! Sometimes we learn the best from our "happy accidents". For these reasons I do not believe in "spoon feeding" people or dictating exact amounts of ingredients.

To me, every meal is like a piece of art. I do not mean that everything we make needs to be gorgeous and impeccably presented, with a perfect blend of colors, etc. Instead, what I mean is that each meal is a work of improvisation- with slight variations due each time to what ingredients you have on hand, your mood or appetite at the moment, what is seasonable and appropriate to the time of year or climate, your personal taste preferences, etc. If you learn to prepare food this way, then I really think you will start to have more fun with your food and begin to have a more enjoyable and healthier relationship with food.

One of the keys to success is having the right tools on hand. Every mechanic needs the right tools and so does every artist. This is equally true in the kitchen. Fortunately, you don't need much to be a nutrient-dense artist. In addition to the basics- some good cookware including decent skillets and pots and pans, I also strongly recommend you have two additional main tools- a good blender, and a good juicer. Both will come in handy and should become highly appreciated, frequently used appliances.

As you will see, nutrient-dense eating relies less on pre-packaged mixes and more on creating meals from "scratch". If you have a diversity of fresh food on hand, then preparing a meal on the spur of the moment is easy! My "meals" tend to be really simple- usually I just throw together whatever is on hand and whatever I am in the mood for. Elaborate meals with lots of ingredients and a lot of time consuming measuring and preparation is usually not only unnecessary but often less rewarding then a simple, down-to-earth yet elegant dish. **My basic rules of thumb are: keep it simple, keep it healthy, keep it delicious.** If you follow these three rules, you can't go wrong!

Some Nutrient-Dense Breakfast Suggestions

Here is a heads up: nutritious breakfasts are easy! Many of us are super rushed in the mornings, getting ready for work- or getting the kids fed and ready for school- so this is often a time of day when a healthy morning meal gets neglected or sacrificed. This is a shame, because getting some good nourishment into us early in our day is really a crucially important time to send our bodies a message of nutritional support and love. As you will see, a healthy breakfast can be quick, easy, simple, and highly nourishing. Forget the highly processed refined carbohydrate cereals, milk, waffles, breakfast pastries and muffins or doughnuts!

Eggs

Eggs are a perfect nutrient-dense food and a great way to start the day- but only if they are truly free-range and certified organic. Healthy eggs are full of good lipids, lecithin, B vitamins, vitamin A, and protein along with healthy cholesterol- an important nutrient that our nervous systems require to function optimally. Unfortunately many of us have been taught to be "afraid" of eggs- because (so we are told) the cholesterol will cause heart disease. If you prepare your eggs the way I recommend, cholesterol will be your good friend and not your enemy! We actually need cholesterol- we make our favorite hormones- progesterone, estrogen, and testosterone- out of cholesterol in addition to our anti-stress corticosteroid hormones. The key is to not damage the cholesterol – a process called oxidation-which occurs when we burn or over cook it. Excessive heat such as from frying will damage cholesterol and it is this damaged cholesterol that is bad for us. But in its healthy undamaged state cholesterol is an incredibly important nutrient. To preserve cholesterol in its "good" form, cook your eggs at a lower temperature. Instead of frying your eggs, boil them. Poaching and hard or soft-boiled eggs are a great way to enjoy them and get the benefits without the worry

Recommended Breakfast Options

- **Breakfast Option** 2-3 organic free-range eggs poached, soft boiled, or hard boiled. Nutrient-dense suggestions: drizzle with flax oil; a pinch of mineral rich sea salt, pepper, cayenne, nutritional yeast, powdered kelp or dulse. Eat alone, or with a slice of nutrient-dense toast- spread toast with coconut oil. Add a wedge of avocado.

- **Breakfast Option** Glass of fresh juice straight from your juicer. There are whole books of recipes or use your imagination. My standard juice recipe base usually consists of several carrots (depends upon their size), a half apple, a fingertip size piece of fresh ginger root, and a quarter lemon. If you want something a bit "heartier" add ¼ or ½ fresh beet, a stalk or two of celery and/or 1/3 or so of a fresh cucumber. Adjust the proportions to get the taste you like the best- juicing is an "improvisational art" so have fun and enjoy!

- **Breakfast Option** Slice or two of gluten-free or nutrient-dense toast (see appendix for "best breads") and spread with coconut oil and/or almond butter. Option: sprinkle some cinnamon (good for blood sugar issues), top with some sliced fresh apple or fresh berries or banana.

- **Breakfast Option** Coconut oil toast (see above) with avocado slices, fresh tomato/red onion. Option: add some sliced olives or capers, hummus, or smoked salmon if you eat fish.

- **Breakfast Option** Fruit Bowl- chopped up fresh fruit medley. Option: toss in a handful of almonds or walnuts. Option: wet it up with a half cup of fresh squeezed orange juice (or take a couple of oranges, minneola, tangerines, etc. and just squeeze the juice over the fruit. Option: sprinkle some unsweetened coconut flakes or shreds into the bowl or a spoonful of Ultra-Dense Breakfast Boost (see smoothie #1, below).

- **Breakfast Option** Have your-self a "Nude Smoothie". There are a couple basic versions- one uses coconut milk or almond milk as a creamy "base", and the other style uses fresh fruit juice for a lighter, fruitier style.

Basic Smoothie #1: In a Nutri-Bullet^{tm} or standard blender add 2 bananas (three if small), some coconut milk or coconut cream, ½ tsp. or more of spirulina powder and a scoop or two of Ultra-Dense Breakfast Boost from Crystal River Organics (see appendix). Blend and enjoy! Options: add some ice if you prefer it to be thicker and colder. Options; cinnamon, vanilla extract, bee pollen, stevia or a little honey, black strap molasses, or, other fruits like frozen or fresh berries instead of the bananas (or, in addition to the bananas).

Basic Smoothie #2 Another option is to make a rich chocolate version adapting the Basic Smoothie #1 recipe but omit the spirulina and substitute a Tbsp. or two of unsweetened cacao powder. For added density add a spoonful of almond butter or organic peanut butter. Great with a spoonful of blackstrap molasses mixed in. Use a scoop of Ultra-Dense Breakfast Boost Coconut-Pecan!

Basic Smoothie #3 Substitute a fresh juice like squeezed orange juice in place of the coconut milk. Use a variety of berries with or without some banana. This version is best with the Ultra-Dense Berry Blend flavor.

Note: the above breakfast options present a wide variety of ways to start your day. Since everyone is different, you might experiment with several of these to see what suits your particular body and metabolism the best. Some of these breakfast options are higher in carbs, some are higher in protein, and some are more balanced or neutral- but all are nutrient-dense and delicious!

Mid-Morning Snack Options

It's interesting how so many people's blood sugar crashes in the mid-morning- most likely this is due to too many refined carbohydrates first thing in the morning. Plus that's the time the earlier coffee kick crashes for many of us! The best solution is a more nutrient-dense breakfast- any of the above breakfast options should really help. The important thing is to listen to your body- it is far better to snack throughout the day with small nutrient-dense "mini-meals" that keep nourishing your body (as opposed to just giving it more empty calories). This is a smart way to keep your metabolism supported.

If your workplace has a refrigerator, keep several key items handy- a bottle of flax oil, umeboshi plum vinegar, a container of hummus. Why not take a five minute snack break with something healthy that you can throw together yourself instead of relying on the vending machine or other convenient- but not so healthy choices?

Try fueling your metabolic fire with some of the following mid-morning snack options:

- **Morning Snack Option:** try a Nude Food Bar (see appendix for information) from Crystal River Organics

- **Morning Snack Option:** Fresh fruit; 1 or 2 medium size bananas will fill you up or try peeling an orange or two.

- **Morning Snack Option:** Fresh glass of live juice

- **Morning Snack Option:** 1-2 Hard-boiled eggs

- **Morning Snack Option:** Handful or two of raw, unroasted almonds

- **Morning Snack Option:** Cup of green tea, mate, kombucha

- **Morning Snack Option:** spoonful or two of almond butter; spread some on some celery stalks or a rice cake

- **Morning Snack Option:** Smoothie! Either finish the one from your breakfast (I recommend getting a good quality thermos) or make a fresh one.

A Healthy Appetite

Don't worry if you get ravenously hungry when transitioning to a more nutrient-dense diet between meals- a strong appetite is a good sign that your metabolism is revving up and looking for some healthy fuel. Many people hardly ever experience a strong appetite- they just eat according to the clock, or out of boredom, or for other reasons (such as when they feel depressed and are looking for comfort food, etc). Eating this way can actually suppress the arising of "real" hunger. If you do experience strong "body" hunger, as opposed to "psychological" hunger, then you are on the right track. Often many of us reach for a snack (usually something fairly unhealthy) at the slightest twinge of hunger, and never give a stronger hunger time to develop. If this is your tendency, then try to hold off for a few minutes and not give in to the first twinge of hunger- often you will discover that much of what we think is hunger is actually a mental state of boredom that we unconsciously try to block out or erase with food.

Lunch Options

Nutrient-dense, metabolism-enhancing lunches are easy and delicious! If you tend to go out for lunch with co-workers, try and find places that serve healthy things like salads, hummus plates and the like. Japanese sushi places are generally a good option. Soups sometimes work well too- *if* they are homemade and don't have a dairy (milk/cream) base and don't use non-organic animal meat. Remember, burgers, chicken, and pizza are out unless you have an unusually healthy place to go to that serves organic meat and cheese (this is getting better in some parts of the country, but unfortunately, this is still extremely rare!). One more tip- if you know you will be going out somewhere and you anticipate ordering a large salad, try bringing your own nutrient-dense dressing! I will be giving you a couple of great recipe ideas below that I guarantee will be more nutrient-dense and more delicious than anything that will be served with lunch!

- **Lunch Option:** Sardines on bed of lettuce placed on gluten-free toast or rice cakes. Top with diced red onion or olives. Side of avocado, fresh tomato, carrot, and/or celery sticks

- **Lunch Option:** Super Salad with homemade nutrient-dense dressing

- **Lunch Option:** Super Soup

- **Lunch Option:** Hard-boiled eggs and vegetables. Dip veggies in salad dressing (recipes below)Option: Devilled eggs (recipe below)

- **Lunch Option:** Leftover dinner entrée.

- **Lunch Option:** Ultra-Dense Smoothie

- **Lunch Option:** Mediterranean plate: Hummus/olives/avocado/carrot, celery, grape tomatoes, dolmas (rice with olive oil and fresh herbs wrapped in a grape leaf), salsa

- **Lunch Option:** Almond butter sandwich with mashed banana, cinnamon, raisins on nutrient-dense bread or rice cakes

- **Lunch Option:** Hummus, avocado, alfalfa sprouts open face on rice cake(s). Drizzle a little flax seed oil on top and sprinkle a few drops of umeboshi plum vinegar

- **Lunch Option:** Buffalo burger- without the bun. Serve with plenty of salad greens, sliced tomato, red onion. Drizzle with flax oil, a splash of umeboshi plum vinegar, or spice it up with some cayenne!

Easy Dinner Options

"What's for dinner?" is often a perennial refrain at most homes. Whether you are cooking for one, two, or for an entire family, throwing together a quick and nutritious dinner is a surprising snap once you learn a few basics. I've learned how to become a master at quick skillet dinners and stir fries and you can find additional recipes and tips on www.thenutrientsmartdiet.com – they are surprisingly fast- and a real bonus is that there is always very little to clean up! Make enough so there will be leftovers-this is a great way to get at least two meals out of one prep. Also make it a habit to always have a large nutrient-dense salad with a fresh nutrient-dense dressing (see Salad dressing section, below) as an integral part of most of your dinner meals.

Gluten-Free Whole Grains

Learning to cook whole grains- specifically brown rice, millet and quinoa- is an important and useful skill. Although many are intimidated at the idea, these whole grains are nutritious and actually super easy to cook. Be fearless and your learning curve will be short and painless! Whole grains are a great staple for many nutrient-dense meals, and provide good nutrition at an inexpensive price. Make extra for the next day or two as a convenient way to have extra food on hand for a quick meal or snack. I use all three of these grains as staples in a variety of ways- from stir-fries to rice/lentil stews to soups to a breakfast accompaniment with eggs and more.

Dinner Options

- **Dinner Option:** Buffalo Skillet Stir-Fry with brown rice

- **Dinner Option:** Wild Salmon with mixed vegetables and quinoa

- **Dinner Option:** Tempeh Skillet dish- with rice, millet, or quinoa

- **Dinner Option:** Saag Paneer (non-dairy, made with coconut cream) with brown rice

- **Dinner Option:** Buckwheat soba noodles tossed with mixed vegetables, shiitake mushrooms and tofu

- **Dinner Option:** Steamed Vegetable medley (served with flax oil over brown rice, millet, or quinoa)

- **Dinner Option:** Brown rice/lentil "stew"- basically a very thick hearty "soup" featuring shiitake mushrooms, carrot, onion, celery, broccoli, (and whatever else is in your refrigerator or strikes your fancy). Perfect vehicle for adding flax oil, nutritional yeast, etc.

- **Dinner Option:** Organic tomato sauce spaghetti with spaghetti squash noodles (or with buckwheat soba noodles)
- **Dinner Option:** Hearty nutrient-dense soup with baked yam

- **Dinner Option:** Curried vegetables over rice (add tofu, tempeh, nuts, or other protein if desired)

- **Dinner Option:** Super Salad with all the fixins and homemade nutrient-dense salad dressing.

- **Dinner Option Side dishes:** lightly steamed greens such as beet greens, kale, chard with flax oil drizzle; smashed potatoes (see recipe, below) made with coconut oil and sea salt, side salad, boiled beets, vegetable medley

- **Dinner Option Condiments:** My standards are: nutritional yeast, umeboshi vinegar, salsa, and seaweeds. Use whichever are appropriate to the main dish you are serving.

Dairy-Free Mashed Potatoes

Nutrient-Dense Mashed Potatoes! Who doesn't love mashed potatoes? They can serve as a great comfort food side dish and more. Try this version for a dairy free, more nutrient-dense take on an old favorite: In a large mixing bowl, mash up some well-cooked still warm boiled or baked potatoes (organic, with the skins on please!). I will not give you amounts of the following ingredients because it depends upon how many potatoes and how big a batch you are making. Add in a dollop or two of virgin coconut oil (this replaces dairy butter). Also add in some coconut milk or coconut cream (this replaces ordinary cow's milk) and whisk or whip in for a nice creamy texture. Salt and pepper to taste. Variations: add in some diced celery for texture and crunch and /or fresh herbs like cilantro. A little paprika or turmeric will give the mashed potatoes a nice golden glow. A touch of cayenne can be nice if you like a little heat. You can sprinkle in a dash of powdered kelp or dulse (sea weed) for some extra trace minerals. Another nice variation is to add in some frozen organic peas or corn. The sweetness of the peas or corn makes a nice counterpoint to the savory-ness of the mashed potatoes.

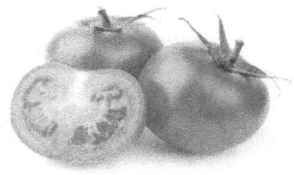

Nutrient-Dense Salad Dressings

Salads are a really important part of a successful nutrient-dense eating plan and an appropriately delicious and nutritious dressing is the perfect complement- both taste-wise as well as from a nutritional point of view. The following recipes will show you how to make your own fresh and delicious dressings that are far tastier and healthier than anything you can buy in a bottle. Once you find a version that you love, you will want to make a large batch and store it in your fridge. Keep some on hand in the refrigerator at work, or find a handy small bottle that you can put in your pocket or handbag when you go to a restaurant so you can have a really healthy salad away from home. These also are great for dipping vegetables!

Umeboshi Plum Vinegar

Umeboshi plums are a traditional Japanese food that is reputed to have strong health- supporting effects. These are small plums that are aged in a brine solution and allowed to naturally ferment. The soft moist salted plums are eaten medicinally as they are considered very alkaline in the macrobiotic tradition. They are also made into a paste which is also used as a delicious condiment. Umeboshi paste and vinegar are very strongly salty, so a little goes a long way! Leaves of the shiso plant are used in the preparation process which gives the plums, paste, and vinegar a beautiful rosy or purplish hue. The plum vinegar is much more salty and is more tart than it is vinegary, and has a fresh, clean, crisp "bright" taste that makes it perfect in salad dressings and as a condiment or flavoring for waking up many dishes.

Salad Dressing #1
The most basic dressing has just two ingredients. But as you will see, it is easy to start adding to this base. Surprisingly delicious! Ingredients: fresh flax oil, umeboshi plum vinegar.

Use just enough flax oil to coat the leaves of the lettuce and other vegetables, and put in a light splash or so of the vinegar and toss. Umeboshi is a light, tart, salty vinegar that gives a bright taste to things. It goes very well with good quality flax oil. Don't overdo the umeboshi- it is quite salty and a little goes a long way. Fresh flax oil (which should always be refrigerated) is a bit stronger tasting compared with ordinary, refined conventional oils so don't overdo it either!

Salad Dressing #2
This one is more complex than #1, but uses the same flax oil/umeboshi vinegar combination as a starting point. In a bottle or jar add: 2-4 oz flax oil, 1-3 Tbsp. umeboshi plum vinegar, 6-8 oz. extra virgin olive oil, a squeeze of lemon juice, ½ tsp powdered kelp or dulse, squirt of organic mustard, dollop of wasabi mayonnaise or vegan substitute. Blend or shake vigorously. Makes approx. 12 oz. of simply awesome dressing! Caution: start slowly with the umeboshi and add a little at a time until you get the right flavor. Don't overdo it!

Salad Dressing #3
Here is another variation that is simply delicious! In a bottle or jar combine:
4 oz. flax oil, 6-8 oz extra virgin olive oil, 1-2 Tbsp. umeboshi vinegar, 1 Tbsp. almond butter, 1 Tbsp. nutritional yeast flakes. Mix or shake vigorously!

Salad Dressing #4
Tahini-lemon dressing! Easy and delicious! In a bowl, bottle or jar combine: 3 Tbsp. tahini (sesame butter), ½ cup extra virgin olive oil- whisk together or blend well, add 2Tbs nutritional yeast, blend in, then add 2-3 Tbsp. fresh flax oil, a pinch of sea

salt, 1 Tbsp. umeboshi plum vinegar, squeeze in a couple tsp. of fresh lemon juice. Blend or whisk all together.

Salad Dressing #5
Honey mustard yumminess! Blend together 1-2 Tbs of good raw honey with 1 Tbs of organic mustard. Blend with 3 oz flax oil and 6-8 oz extra virgin olive oil mixture. Add a dollop of almond butter and mix well. A splash of umeboshi plum vinegar will really enhance the sweet/savory marriage in this dressing
.

Salad Dressing variations: The above recipes all provide "ballpark" proportions and measurements. Rely on your own taste buds and preferences to give your dressing your own personal signature. Some great variations include blending in a ripe avocado to create a creamier "green goddess" effect. Minced or pressed garlic of course is a classic addition for many salad dressings. You can also add in a little of the juice from the olives you purchase from the deli or olive bar- briny olive water is super flavorful and adds a really nice dimension to a dressing. Black pepper is also an important addition to many dressings. Fresh herbs are both nutrient-dense as well as delicious! Whether from the store, a farmer's market, or your own or a neighbor's garden, it's great to add some freshly diced tarragon, cilantro, mint, basil, or oregano. I also like to add some nutritional yeast to many of my dressings- this really boosts the nutritional denseness of the dressing and brings a nice subtle nutty savory-ness to the dressing. A sprinkle of powdered kelp or dulse can also provide more complexity to the finished taste profile as well as contributing trace minerals.

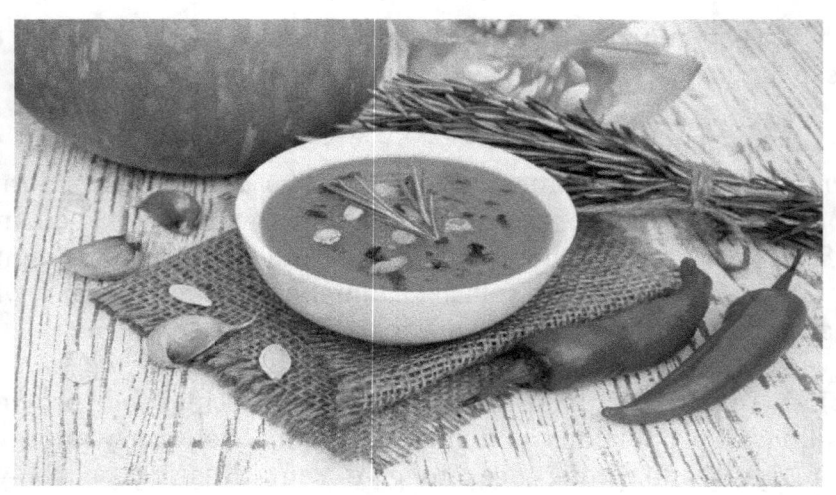

Super Soups

Soups are a wonderful and versatile way to add nutrient-density to your diet. I think of soups as a blank canvass from which great meals can be made. There is virtually no limit to the different combinations and ingredients you can use. Soups can be a great budget-stretcher too. I usually intentionally make too much, so you can enjoy leftovers the next day or two from one meal. If you have a thermos it is easy to take your liquid lunch on the go with you.

Here are some of the many ingredients that work well in many soups: lentils, beans, split peas, all vegetables, plus onion, garlic, etc., mushrooms, frozen organic peas and corn, brown rice, quinoa, or millet, stewed or fresh tomatoes, seaweed, olives, miso, tofu, nutritional yeast, fresh herbs and spices. Coconut cream or coconut milk makes an excellent base for creamy style soups. You can also use rice noodles or buckwheat soba noodles. If you eat meat, a little organic meat or seafood works well too.

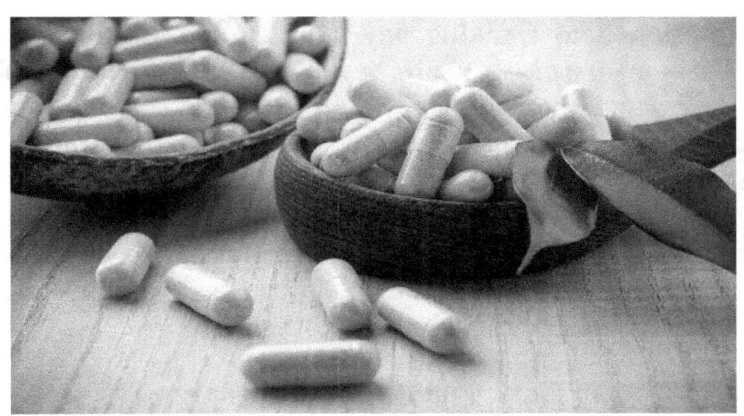

Chapter 13

Specific Supplements for Weight Management

There are many nutrients touted for weight management these days. The truth is, not everything works for everyone, and what doesn't work for you *could* work for someone else (and vice versa). In the end, only first-hand experience-experimental trials- will help you understand how specific nutrients can affect you and help you achieve your weight and health goals.

With this in mind, I am about to introduce you to some very specific nutrients that are known to work directly in the energy producing pathways that we discussed in our chapters on metabolism. Again, I am *not* suggesting everyone should take all of these! Rather, I am offering here an admittedly quick overview of some of my top favorite metabolism-supporting supplements. Research shows that these nutrients are capable of supplying some of the basic biochemical keys to help unlock the stuck metabolic fires that have been damped down within some people's cells. As I said earlier, I recommend you run these by a qualified health care provider who knows your health history and situation before taking any supplements. While generally regarded as extremely safe, everyone is slightly different genetically and biochemically. And if you are taking any medications or prescription drugs, then it is important to make sure that nothing could interfere or react with your meds.

The following are presented in no particular order. Just because I have listed them in this order doesn't mean that the first ones are "better" or more necessary than others.

And please remember, the core of this program is still the nutrient-dense *diet*- this is really a lifetime *eating* plan. Generally speaking, supplements are not intended for long term or lifelong use; rather they can be helpful for jump-starting a really stuck or struggling metabolic situation and helping to nudge your metabolism in the right direction.

The Supplements

Selenium: This is an important mineral for weight loss because **it plays a key role in thyroid hormone activation**. A word of warning- too much selenium can be mildly toxic – however ingesting too much is actually quite rare. Do some research, and then check with your trusted health care professional before taking, especially if you are already on thyroid hormones. A good generally accepted safe dosage range for most adults might be between 50 and 200 mg per day.

Zinc: Zinc is another very important mineral with some highly specific roles to play in how the body processes food. **Zinc is biochemically necessary for the metabolism of most proteins.** Many people take between 25-50 mg per day in the form of zinc chelate or zinc citrate.

Magnesium: Magnesium is vitally important throughout the body and is actively involved in every organ system in the body.

More enzymatic chemical reactions require magnesium than any other mineral. **Magnesium is also essential for energy production in the chain of steps leading to ATP synthesis.** Studies show that most Americans do not get adequate amounts of magnesium from their diets, especially those who eat a lot of highly processed junk foods. Magnesium is also helpful in many cases for jangled nerves, insomnia, and nervous irritability as well as muscle cramps and spasms, asthma, and PMS.

Magnesium is also a very important mineral for cardiovascular health. There are many forms of magnesium available and all are beneficial, but for maximum metabolic support try magnesium citrate either in capsules or as a powder that you can add directly to juice or a smoothie. Dosage depends upon your body size, state of metabolism, dietary habits, etc. Generally accepted safe and effective levels range from 400mg to 1000 mg per day (usually in divided doses). High levels can lead to diarrhea in some individuals so it is best to start slowly and work your way up.

Vitamin C: Vitamin C, or ascorbic acid as it is commonly sold, is a crucial nutrient of major importance to overall health. An important water-soluble antioxidant, vitamin C is always associated in nature with fresh produce- an indicator that it is intimately intended to be a biologically important accompaniment to a plant based diet. Recent studies are showing a close relationship between vitamin C levels and weight. **Recent research has shown that optimal levels of vitamin C increases the rate at which fat is oxidized (metabolized).** *The Nutrient-Dense Diet* certainly strongly recommends eating generous amounts of fresh produce daily- especially fruit- as a way to ensure you are getting all the enzymes, pigments, vitamin C, minerals, fiber, and other nutrients that come with eating raw, unprocessed, fresh foods, such as fresh or recently harvested fruits and vegetables.

A glass of freshly squeezed fruit or citrus juice daily should ensure you are getting adequate amounts, but if you don't eat much fresh fruit, it might be a good idea to take a vitamin C supplement. For weight loss support, I recommend a range with 1000 mg on the low end to several thousand mg on the upper end of the scale, taken in divided doses. Like magnesium, high levels can occasionally lead to diarrhea if you are not used to it, but this is rare.

Essential Fatty Acids: Both the omega-three and omega-six fatty acids are necessary for our health and metabolism to function properly. In particular **cell and mitochondrial membranes work best if essential fatty acids are present-** from fresh food sources. The Standard American Diet typically contains far too many of the omega-six family compared to the threes, so most nutrient-dense diets recommend supplementation with a good quality source of omega-threes to help restore a more balanced ratio. Fish oils such as from cod or salmon, or krill (very small marine plankton- like creatures) are excellent sources and for vegetarians, flax, hemp, and walnut oils are good sources. Buy a reputable brand, and keep refrigerated to protect it after opening as good oils are prone to rancidity.

Carnitine: l-carnitine is an amino acid–like molecule that plays a uniquely important role in fat metabolism. **Carnitine acts like a shuttle, actually transporting fat molecules into the cell where they can be metabolized within the mitochondria for energy.** Carnitine deficiencies are thought by some researchers to be associated with lack of energy, fatigue, and a generally sluggish metabolism which of course can lead to weight gain. Very safe when used as directed, l-carnitine is a strongly recommended component of this program. **Vegetarians might be particularly at risk for not getting enough carnitine**. Vitamin C is also necessary for the body to synthesize carnitine. Recommended safe and effective dosage levels are from 500-2500 mg per day, depending upon the severity of your metabolic bottleneck.

Trace Minerals: Trace minerals may provide a spark that can encourage a sluggish metabolism to rev up. Trace minerals reflect the biochemical diversity of nature and the natural environment. Virtually every mineral on earth is found dissolved in sea water, though typically in ultra-tiny (nano) amounts. Seaweeds are a great way to give your body a little boost of these substances. There are also some good supplements available on the market that provides small but concentrated amounts of trace minerals. Take as directed.

CoQ 10: CoQ10 acts as an antioxidant that supports metabolic efficiency at the mitochondrial level. There is quite a bit of research supporting the important role of this nutrient in promoting cellular metabolic health. **It is believed that 95% of the energy used by the human body depends upon adequate CoQ10 levels.** In order to synthesize it in the body, numerous nutrients are necessary, so any marginal deficiencies in these vitamins could lead to a deficiency in CoQ10 production. It is well known that statin drugs, commonly prescribed to lower cholesterol and for heart disease, dramatically lowers CoQ10 levels.

Pyruvate (Pyruvic Acid): Pyruvate is another interesting molecule that is directly involved in cellular energy production. Pyruvate metabolism occurs in the mitochondria, and is the first real step in the whole Krebs cycle, being produced from the breakdown of glucose. **Weight loss studies have shown that taking 5 grams or so per day is an effective (and safe) dosage.** Interestingly, the richest dietary source of pyruvic acid is red apples!

Ribose: Ribose is a fascinating molecule that is being actively researched for its role in energy production, sports performance, and endurance. Ribose is incorporated into several vital larger molecules including DNA and RNA as well as ATP! A very safe nutrient with little to no negative side effects, **experts recommend taking 2000-6000 mg daily for metabolic support.**

B Vitamins: **The B vitamins are especially important as co-enzymes or facilitators in the Citric Acid Cycle, or Krebs cycle leading to ATP production**. Thiamine (B_1,) , Riboflavin (B_2), and Niacin (B_3) are all crucially important vitamins. Nutritional yeast is a particularly good source of these vitamins. Alcohol (ethanol) destroys B_1.   High consumption of refined carbohydrates increases the need for B vitamins.

Tyrosine: Tyrosine is another extremely important metabolism supporting amino acid. It plays several key roles including being the backbone molecule for thyroid hormone. **It also is the precursor for CoQ10 production**. Tyrosine is known to be helpful in many cases of stress and fatigue.

Creatine: Creatine supports the synthesis and regeneration of ATP. It is used in large amounts by the high-energy demand tissues in the body. In the diet creatine is mainly supplied by meat so vegetarians might be at risk and could possibly benefit from supplementation. **Studies have shown that Creatine can measurably improve muscle contraction and strength**. Five to twenty grams a day have been safely used in studies and by many consumers, including athletes and bodybuilders.

A Final Word about Supplements

Please remember- supplements are not a "magic bullet". They are just what the word means- supplements- meaning they are intended to be adjuncts to our diet- not the main course! As a society we have become very reliant on drugs of all kinds and tend to regard many pills and supplements as the quick fix answer to our needs.

None of the supplements mentioned will unlock your stuck metabolism all by themselves and lead to effortless weight loss. Rather they will likely work best as synergistic nutrients in conjunction with other nutrients and in combination with a nutrient-dense diet. Remember, metabolic issues tend to be fairly complex and often involve multiple problems that need to be solved over time. Keep your expectations in check and take supplements responsibly and they can be a valuable ally and aid in your weight loss program.

Chapter 14

Summary of the Nutrient-Dense Diet Program

Let's take a moment now and summarize the Nutrient-Dense Diet program. Instead of throwing together a lot of unrelated pieces, we can now begin to see that there is really one nice, unified vision of health here. This is a healthy lifestyle, rooted in common sense and utilizing a comprehensive selection of healthy habits that reinforce the message of good health- all with the goal of supporting, strengthening and enhancing cellular metabolic functioning.

Summary

- **Drink lots of water; and make sure it is high quality water- chlorine and fluoride are both metabolic poisons. Avoid plastic where possible.**

- **Move your body more; exercise, walk, move, stretch. Do yoga.**

- **Breathe gently and always through your nose.**

- **Avoid junk food; especially avoid empty-calorie junk foods. No chips, fried foods, candy; and strictly limit, or better yet eliminate entirely breads, pastries, cookies, and the like. Absolutely no NutraSweet (Aspartame) containing products. If you use a lot of salt, please cut back. Too much salt can adversely affect metabolic functioning by upsetting the balance of fluids and electrolytes in your body and cells and cause water retention.**

141

- **Eat lots of (or only) nutrient-dense foods. Enjoy all the fresh fruit and vegetables you want. Use only organic meats and cheeses. Organic eggs are very nutrient-dense, especially if they are boiled or poached.. If you are not allergic, eat plenty of unroasted nuts and seeds. They are full of good oils, fiber, vitamins, and minerals. Fresh juices are your best friend! Prepare (juice) them fresh and drink as frequently as possible. Buy and eat berries galore- fresh is best but frozen are fine too. Add as many of the following as possible and learn how to integrate these into your diet: herb teas, whole grains such as millet, brown rice, quinoa; use flax seed oil liberally for salad dressings and only as a cold oil, and use coconut butter, especially when you need to sauté, bake, or gently fry something. Incorporate superfoods such as seaweeds, spirulina, bee pollen, nutritional yeast, umeboshi plum paste and lots of spices and herbs including turmeric, cinnamon and cayenne. Eat lots of salads. If you can find it give raw goat milk a try. Nut butters, such as almond butter are great; check out almond milk as well.**

- **Take the suggested metabolism supporting supplements that are right for you.**

- **Think and act positively! Work on handling your stress. We all have some!**

- **Believe in yourself!!**

Basically that is it. If you follow the above advice you should see and feel rather dramatic results. In other words, if you really get more exercise, drink water daily, avoid or drastically cut back on the junk, eat NuDe (nutrient-densely), and take the recommended supplements, your body will transform from what you have now to a much healthier, happier you. I would be greatly surprised if you didn't have more energy, a leaner, more fit body, more enthusiasm, more motivation, and more creativity than before starting the program. And most importantly, instead of a quick fix, you will have learned the skills necessary to live healthily for the rest of your life.

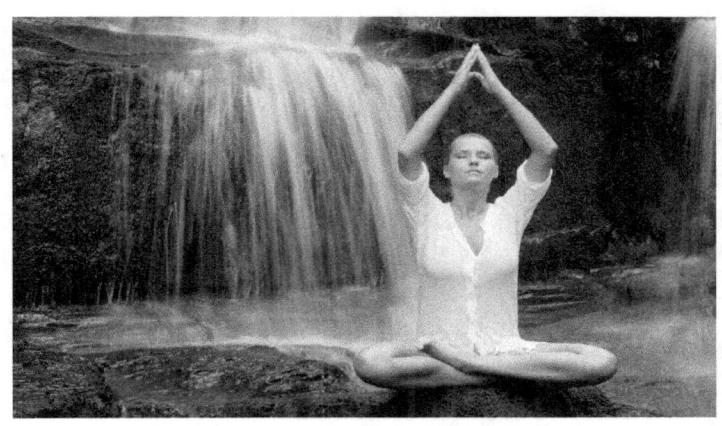

Chapter 15

The **NuDe** you!
Celebrating Your **Individuality**

Your weight management program is for *you!* The good news about cellular dormancy is that each person has slightly different reasons for his or her metabolic situation as well as its severity. And that means that each person's solution will be slightly different as well. **This means that your optimal weight loss program and eating style should be unique to you**. Your tastes, your lifestyle, your preferences, your family, your home, and your schedule are all different from everyone else's and so too will be your personal approach to adopting a nutrient-dense lifestyle.

Nutrient-density *works*. Improving your diet in profound and substantial ways cannot help but increase the efficiency of your metabolic biochemistry. What nutrient-density has going for it, is science- and common sense. It is *intuitively* right and it is scientifically valid. By treating your body with respect- by supplying your body with the most generous amounts of all the vital elements of nutrition, your body cannot help but come into its own true balance. And the bottom line is that it is only through balance that your body can achieve permanent and safe weight loss.

Equally obvious and intuitively true is that the SAD diet cannot possibly build sustainable, lasting, great health. Artificial, synthetic, foreign-to-the-body chemicals and GMOs that frequently mimic and confuse the body's natural systems are inimical to health. At the very least, our bodies have to expend vitally needed energy just to identify and deal with these substances. At worst, many of these chemicals and other toxins may strongly interfere with our metabolic machinery, and may trigger various imbalances, resulting in physiological stress, and leading or contributing to diseases including such modern epidemics as some forms of cancer, and of course, obesity.

A nutrient-dense diet can look like just about anything you can imagine. This means that you can be vegetarian and have a nutrient-dense diet or have carnivorous habits and be nutrient-dense. You can eat cooked food and be nutrient-dense or you can eat a raw, live diet and be nutrient-dense. And you can eat gluten and still be nutrient-dense or you can be gluten-free and be nutrient-dense. The only practical approach is to understand there needs to be a tremendous amount of flexibility among healthy diets to accommodate people's diverse tastes.

 Allow your diet to stay innovative and flexible while remaining consistent to nutrient-dense principles by ingesting a wide range of exceptionally nutrient-dense foods, and you can't go wrong. Using a nutrient-dense diet in order to improve your cellular functioning is the only sensible way to honor your body and its uniqueness.

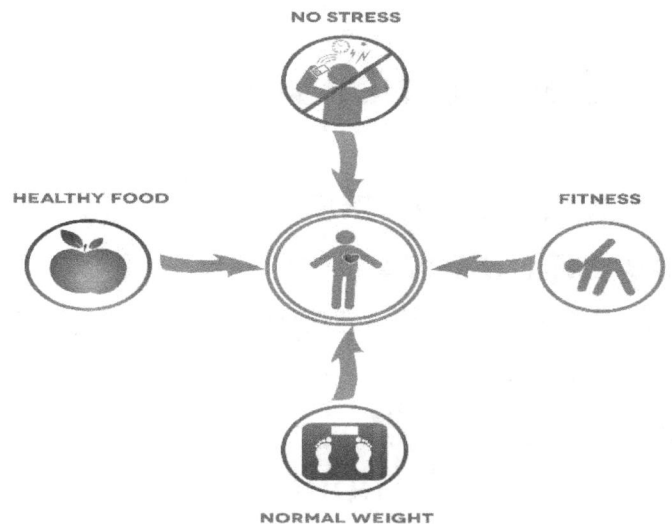

Holistic
Weight Management

Many people think that weight management has just one goal- to achieve (and then maintain) their desired weight target. But a truly *holistic* approach offers much more than just weight loss. In fact, many weight management programs are unable to achieve *lasting* weight loss because they don't address the underlying issues that often accompany weight gain and poor physical health. Having comprehensive, holistic goals is the nutrient-smart difference!

Comprehensive Goals

- Lose weight relatively easily and permanently
- Have more energy and enthusiasm about life
- Feel better about oneself
- Feel more in control of one's life
- Feel more hopeful about the future
- Develop more self-confidence
- Develop more awareness about one's body and health
- Feel more confident about food choices and options
- Learn new cooking and food preparation skills
- Learn how to nourish and help loved ones
- Understand how food is grown and raised and how our food choices affect the environment and world around us.

Final Thoughts

A successful weight loss program is based on several key ingredients. First, the program itself needs to be intelligent, scientifically sound, and understandable. Secondly, the person who is following it needs to ...well, follow it! **This basically means having the sincere inspiration, motivation, and persistence to put it into practice and to apply the principles on a consistent, day-to-day basis.** Doing the "one step forward, one step back" dance will not yield significant results nor very good progress. Remember, if you are after a true lifestyle change, then you have to change your lifestyle! This means leaving the old, unhealthy lifestyle behind and making friends with your new lifestyle and identity. You can't have it both ways! So **being decisive about your decision to lose weight and become healthier is perhaps the most important thing of all.**

The other key components needed for success are (1) will power, (2) patience, and (3) the right strategies to make the process easier and enjoyable. On most paths we should expect to encounter occasional rough patches or challenging situations. Not all journeys are 100% smooth sailing! Having a set of core strategies can help us ride out the waves during the inevitable bumpy moments when things get a bit challenging and we are tempted to cheat or quit.

Throwing in the towel prematurely is a real shame- especially when things are starting to go well. Sometimes we can't always see that things are metabolically improving- especially early on- and our personal frustration and unrealistic expectations can occasionally get in the way of our longer term success. Remember, your scale in the bathroom is not the only indicator of how well you are doing!

Final Secrets

So now I will divulge my parting thoughts and my final top secrets about weight loss- and any other positive change you may want to make in your life. These are the secret keys that can separate success from failure-shhhh- please keep these to yourself, or only share these with those who are ready to hear these special tips!

Decisiveness- Your personal inner drive and ambition. Everything else follows this. Once you make the decision to undertake a major change or set a goal for yourself, the big question is how badly and sincerely you really want it. You have to mean it! If you are wishy-washy, casual, or lackadaisical about your goals, there is an excellent chance you won't achieve them! Be firmly decisive in setting your goals- this is the first step and it is vital to get off on the right foot!

Determination- Think of it as your "inner bulldog". How persistent can you be when challenges arise (they will!) and your willpower or inspiration begins to waver?

Anticipation- The ability to look ahead and realistically plan for challenges is a most important key to success. Being able to anticipate that things will not always be simple, straightforward and easy is a sign of maturity and wisdom. Things won't always go smoothly- so the big question is, can you plan for some of the challenges that might arise? What if you are suddenly invited to a restaurant and there is little that is nutrient-dense on the menu? What if there is nothing healthy in your home or apartment and the only apparent option is the convenience store down the street? What if you are on vacation or visiting relatives? If you can anticipate that certain situations might really test your nutrient-dense lifestyle, then hopefully you will be able to improvise and not fall off the wagon too hard (or at all). This is really about learning the fine art of becoming more "proactive" and assertive with regards to your personal health and goals.

Stress Reduction and Relaxation- The biggest threat to our way of life doesn't come from terrorists or any other outside danger. The biggest threat to our happiness comes from- ourselves! Stress, worry, and anxiety are the robbers who steal away our peace of mind and our inner sense of contentment and happiness. Many of us are so caught up in the fast pace of our lives these days that we sometimes forget the simple pleasures and joys of life. When we are under a lot of stress we can even forget that life is to be valued and enjoyed!

On a purely physiological level we know that stress causes the release of hormones that can accelerate aging, suppress our immune system, depress our metabolism, and lead to weight gain. Chronic stress, worry, and anxiety not only decrease our happiness but they have been conclusively shown to shorten our lives as well. Stress lowers our quantity of life as well as the quality of it.

Dealing with stressful situations doesn't have to be so hard! In fact it should be fun- but of course, stress is our grouchy old inner self who doesn't want to have a good time-which is why she is so grouchy! The list of potential stress-busters is endless. Take a hot bath. Take a walk in the park. Take up painting or a ceramic class. Join a gym. Take a sauna. Visit a friend, volunteer for something important to you, take a beginners yoga class, get a pet or a fish tank. Breathe. Meditate. Pray. Take some quality time away from the computer. Read a book. Garden. Help a neighbor with a project. Go to a concert or museum or planetarium. Take a drive or walk out into the country. Whatever works for you, and whatever gives you real joy and pleasure-remember- you deserve it! A lot of us get into trouble because we frequently "stress eat"- which is not the best way to deal with stress! So find some healthier ways and smile more!

Congratulations!

You have now discovered the secret keys to unlocking cellular dormancy and to achieving lasting weight loss. I wish you all the luck and success in the world! I sincerely hope you have fun with your new adventure and find the vitality, energy, and passion to make the world a little bit of a better place.

Appendix

Organic vs. Non-Organic?

A lot of folks have the same question when they think about the transition to a more and more nutrient-dense diet. "Do I have to buy everything organic?" This is a very sensible and reasonable question!

Some foods matter more than others in terms of the importance of buying organic. If you are on a limited budget than obviously it is very important to monitor your grocery budget carefully-which probably means you will not be purchasing all organic items. Fortunately it is not necessary to be 100% organic. A few tips and suggestions might make your shopping decisions a bit simpler. Here are my top suggestions:

Certain foods are grown or raised with higher levels of pesticides, etc. than others. Those are the foods where I personally will only buy organic.

Some of the foods that are most important to purchase organically are potatoes, mushrooms, citrus fruit, grapes and raisins, pineapples and a lot of soft fruits, including melons and strawberries. This is because these crops in particular are known to be heavily sprayed. Corn is also important to buy organically because virtually all of the non-organic corn in this country is now GMO. In fact, corn, sugar beets and soy are the main GMO foods today but there are many others and their numbers are growing.

The animal industry is especially bad-and therefore all animal products need to be organic- including all milk, ice cream, yogurt, and cheese! This is because of the widespread use of chemicals including antibiotics and estrogenic hormones and because of the horrendous conditions the animals tend to be raised in. Both of these factors lead to stress, disease, and suffering on an unprecedented scale. Please do not support such practices – remember, you are what you eat! This goes for all meat- poultry, pork, and beef as well as dairy and eggs. And remember, even organically raised animals can suffer horribly. If possible, try and know where your food comes from- especially your meat and animal products.

Knowledge is power, so please realize you can do your part to help the animals and responsible farmers with your purchasing dollars. You can make a difference in your own life as well as in the lives of others if you vote with your dollars wisely!

Best Breads

I admit it- I love bread. And if you are like most people, you do too. But guess what? Most of the bread and other baked products out there are simply not very nutrient-dense. In fact The Nutrient-Dense Diet basically recommends that you avoid virtually all baked products while you are trying to jump-start and improve your metabolic functioning.

On the other hand, for those who are transitioning more slowly towards increasing nutrient-density, there is still room for a little bit of bread- if you use the right brands. Sometimes bread can be quite useful as a vehicle for other nutrient-dense foods such as almond butter, hummus, flax oil, egg salad, sardines, etc. A quick nutrient-dense sandwich can be a useful meal or snack.

The important thing to keep in mind is that there is a large spectrum of quality and dense-ness to choose from. To be honest, 98% of the breads sold commercially are really not very good from a nutrient-dense perspective. Many have added sugars such as high fructose corn syrup and other fillers, preservatives, dough conditioners and other chemicals that may not support optimal metabolic functioning. And most flours are also not very high on the nutrient-dense scale in general.

And then of course, there is the gluten issue. Gluten is a metabolic no-no for many, and for others, it is probably best to keep it limited if not eliminated entirely. So, what are the best breads?

Although there are undoubtedly many very good local "artisanal" bakeries, I have reserved for my list three companies that can be found in most health food stores as well as some of the more mainstream stores coast to coast.

The first brand that I like a lot is called Alvarado St Bakery. They specialize in vegan and sprouted whole grain breads as well as bagels, tortillas, buns and other items. They also have some

157

gluten-free options as well and are quite delicious. These breads have a consistency more like conventional breads, which is quite an achievement since they don't use flour at all- only sprouted rye, wheat, and other grains. Sprouting is thought to increase the levels of certain enzymes and proteins, so this is considered a more nutritious option compared to standard breads made from flour. Go to their website at www.alvaradostreetbakery.com for more information.

The next brand I would like to tell you about is called Food For Life (www.foodforlife.com). They make some really tasty gluten-free breads and other products. All of their products are vegan too- so they are dairy-free as well as egg-free. Like Alvarado St Bakery, Food For Life also has sprouted whole grain breads and other baked products. Their line of dense gluten-free breads are usually found in the freezer case and use ingredients such as nutrient-dense brown rice flour and almond flour. Their bread is best toasted, which brings out the natural sweetness. It is delicious toasted with   coconut oil and almond butter.

Finally, another brand I really like are the Genuine Bavarian Breads that are imported from Germany. These are super dense, thinly sliced breads "baked with mountain spring water". Like the other brands, Bavarian bread is flourless, dense and delicious and comes in eight varieties including Rye, Pumpernickel, Multigrain, Sunflower, Flax seed, and their new Gluten-free Whole Grain version. They are all wonderfully dense and chewy, and like the Food For Life Gluten-free breads, best when toasted to bring out the sweetness. Their website is www.healthygermanbread.com.

Joys of Juicing

Juicing is one of the very best ways to get concentrated nutrients in a delicious convenient form. A good juicer will extract the juice - the "life blood" of fruits and vegetables so your body can quickly absorb the nutrients. Fresh juice is full of the plant's enzymes- small molecules that are only found in "live" or "raw" (i.e. uncooked) foods. This understanding is one of the main principles behind the philosophy of eating a "live" or "raw" food diet. A good juicer is one of the few pieces of "special" equipment needed if you truly want to follow a nutrient-dense lifestyle. Juicing is easy, and can make a big difference to your sense of well-being if you incorporate it into your eating lifestyle on a regular basis. Carrots, celery, beets, ginger and cucumbers are some of the easy, commonly used vegetables along with leafy greens such as kale and spinach. Fruit is easily juiced as well and provides enjoyable, refreshing concentrated nutrition by the glassful. If you like, throw some of the pulp (fiber) back in to get additional benefits. The leftover pulp also makes great compost for your garden!

Basic Juice Recipe

Here is my basic juice recipe:
3-6 carrots (it all depends upon the size of the carrots)
1-2 stalks of celery
½ cucumber
½ apple
¼ lemon
a small piece of fresh ginger root
¼ fresh beet root

Change the proportions and ingredients depending upon your taste buds, produce availability, etc.

Homemade Almond Milk

Homemade almond milk is easy, delicious, and more nutritious than the stuff you buy in boxes from the store. It is also versatile and easy to use- put it in your tea or coffee, or use it in your smoothies or in some oatmeal or drink it straight, perhaps with a little blackstrap molasses stirred in for extra nutrients and sweetness.

Almond milk recipe: soak a handful or two of raw almonds overnight in a bowl of cold water. In the morning pour off the water and put the soaked almonds into a blender or Vitamix with enough fresh cold water to cover the almonds and make a nice milk. Whiz until done. Strain with a cheesecloth or tea strainer if you prefer it thinner or use as is without straining. By varying the amount of water you can have a thinner milk or a richer "cream" consistency. If you desire a little sweetness throw a couple of pitted mejool dates into the blender along with the almonds and water. Other nice options are a splash of vanilla extract or a dash of cinnamon.

Nutrient-Dense Egg Salad
And Devilled Eggs

Egg salad can make a great snack or lunch option. Eggs are a super nutrient-dense food that provides numerous nutrients from protein, to good fats and healthy cholesterol to vitamin A to the mineral sulfur. However it is really important to get healthy "clean" eggs from certified organic, free-range hens. Commercial eggs are highly contaminated with antibiotic and hormone residues- please do <u>not</u> eat them! Here is a great way to "nutrify" ordinary egg salad and transform it into a more nutrient-dense version. Eat it by itself, by the spoonful, or on rice cakes or on gluten free or nutrient-dense bread or toast anytime of the day. This is highly nutritious and great for your metabolism so give it a go!

Note: these are very general, approximate, "ballpark" amounts- adjust the amounts by listening to your own taste buds. The important thing is the *quality* of what is used, not how much!

> 4-6 free range, hard boiled eggs, peeled.
> 2-3 Tbs fresh flax seed oil
> 1 tsp organic mustard
> dash or two of sea salt
> dash black pepper
> 1 Tbs nutritional yeast (optional) note: nutritional yeast
> has a strong taste for some people; if you love it, use more,
> if you hate it, omit it entirely!
> 1 celery stalk, finely diced
> 1 -2 Tbs of red onion, finely diced

Mix all ingredients and mash it up! The main difference between this egg salad and most ordinary ones is that we are substituting fresh flax oil for the less healthy mayonnaise that is typically used. If your egg salad is too dry, add more flax oil, or a dash of extra virgin olive oil.

161

Variations: mix in some chopped pitted olives and/or capers. A dash of cayenne will warm it up if you like heat. If you are adventurous, a little wasabi powder makes a delicious change of pace. Finally, a sprinkling of dark purple dulse flakes adds beautiful sparkles of color, taste, and nutrition.

Note: for devilled eggs, essentially do the same as above but slice the eggs in half length-wise. Separate the yolks and add the oil, mustard, salt, and pepper to the yolks and mash until smooth. Then fill in the egg white "boats". Sprinkle a little paprika or turmeric on top for a "traditional" look or some deep purple dulse flakes for a nice effect.

Nude Food

Crystal River Organics is a natural food company based in Boulder Colorado that makes some great nutrient-dense foods. Their "Nude Food" bars are quite nutrient-dense and delicious and come in six flavors. They are bigger and denser than most bars and have no empty-calorie fillers.

They also make a wonderful smoothie "add-in" called Ultra-Dense Breakfast Boost which is perfect in smoothies as well as stirred into organic yogurt or even mixed in some applesauce or added to oatmeal. Ultra-Dense comes in three versions: An "Original" that is unsweetened and contains spirulina, a "Berry Blend" which is perfect for fruit smoothies, and "Coconut-Pecan" which includes probiotics. Everything they make is gluten-free and vegan. Their website is www.nudefood.com

The Nutrient-Smart Program

The Nutrient-Dense Diet explains the theory and science behind losing weight through metabolic optimization. If you want more information about our weight loss program please go to www.thenutrientsmartdiet.com. The Nutrient-Smart Program uses the principles and ideas from The Nutrient-Dense Diet to help people lose weight safely and effectively. Our website will give you additional, up-to-date information on weight loss and metabolism as well as links to other sites, a shopping cart with nutrient-dense foods and supplements, recipes, a future membership opportunity and much more.

Glossary

Amino Acids- the building blocks or "sub-units" that link together to make larger molecules called proteins. Most amino acids contain nitrogen, but a few contain sulfur. Amino acids are nutrients that must be supplied by the diet.

Anti-Oxidants- molecules that help neutralize or soak up free radicals. Examples are vitamin C, vitamin E, Lipoic acid, bioflavonoids and others.

Ascorbic Acid- another name for vitamin C.

Aspartame- the artificial sweetener with the trade name "NutraSweet^{tm}".

ATP- shorthand for the molecule, Adenosine Tri-Phosphate. ATP is the main energy source in the body, and is produced in every cell within the mitochondria.

Bee pollen- flower pollen collected by honey bees. Considered a very healthy, nutrient-dense "super food".

Cellular dormancy- the condition of metabolic slowing down where the cells have reduced energy production or efficiency of converting carbohydrates and other food molecules into energy.

Cellular respiration- the biochemical chain reaction which involves a transfer of electrons (the electron transfer chain or ETC). This occurs within the Citric Acid Cycle leading to ATP production.

Chlorella- a small blue-green algae, consumed as a nutritious "super food", often in smoothies.

Citric Acid Cycle- also known as the "Krebs cycle". This is the primary cellular energy producing pathway within the mitochondria.

Co-enzymes- co-enzymes work to activate enzymes within the biochemical pathways in the body. Most co-enzymes are either vitamins or minerals.

Empty Calories- calories that do not also contribute vitamins, minerals, or other nutrients. White flour, white rice, white sugar, and alcohol are the main sources of empty calories (see, S.A.D.)

Essential Fatty Acids (EFAs)- essential fatty acids are the nutritionally valuable portion of fats and oils (see: lipids). Omega 3s and omega 6s are the main sources.

Free radicals- these are electron-unbalanced atoms that are highly unstable. They may "attack" nearby atoms in a search for available electrons, which can break down other nearby molecules, leading to damage, inflammation, etc. They are neutralized by anti-oxidants.

Genome- another name for the inherited genetic legacy of an organism.

Gluten- a protein commonly found in wheat, rye, barley and some other grains. Gluten is a common dietary irritant in genetically susceptible individuals.

Krebs cycle- see Citric Acid Cycle.

Lipids- fats and oils

Metabolism- the sum total of all the biochemical reactions in living organisms.

Mitochondria- the "batteries" or power stations within virtually every cell in the body. Energy production and the combustion of food molecules occurs within these.

Monosodium glutamate (MSG)- the most common food additive world-wide. MSG intensifies the perception of flavors and taste in the brain. Classified as an "excitotoxin", many people are sensitive to MSG without even knowing it. Present in the vast majority of processed foods and often not labeled.

Nude, NuDe- abbreviation for "nutrient-dense".

Nutrient-Dense- refers to foods that are concentrated sources of specific nutrients. The opposite of empty calories.

Nutrient-Smart Program- an online program designed to use the principles of "unlocking cellular dormancy" and nutrient-density to facilitate weight loss. www.thenutrientsmartdiet.com

Nutritional Yeast- a specific variety of yeast that is grown and dehydrated for use as a food supplement or condiment. Nutritional yeast is a highly nutrient-dense "super food" and is an excellent source of B vitamins, chromium, selenium, nucleic acids and amino acids.

Omega- three fatty acids- this is a group of important essential fatty acids that have anti-inflammatory properties. Food sources include flax oil, hemp, walnuts, and cold water fish.

Progestins- any of the pharmaceutical versions of natural progesterone.

Protein- large molecules that are made of linked together amino acids. Proteins are rich in nitrogen, and are dietarily important because they are the body's only source of essential amino acids which are re-assembled to create the bodies' many proteins
S.A.D. (Standard American Diet)- the "typical" diet of many Americans, characterized by a lot of fast food, processed food, and empty calories.

Sea weeds- also known as "sea vegetables". Traditionally used by coastal people around the world, sea weeds are useful sources of trace minerals and other phytonutrients. Some common examples include arame, dulse, kelp, kombu, laver, nori, and wakame.

Spirulina- a unique nutrient-dense blue-green algae "super food".

Statins- a class of commonly prescribed pharmaceutical drugs principally designed to lower cholesterol levels. Statins may interfere with cellular metabolism because they are well known to lower Co Q 10 levels.

Super Foods- refers to especially unique, nutrient-dense foods. Examples are bee pollen, cacao, flax oil, nutritional yeast, spirulina, sprouts, and others.

Umeboshi- a Japanese salted, fermented plum. Traditionally used as a macrobiotic food. Can be used as a condiment in paste form or as a vinegar. Considered to be alkaline and nourishing.

D. Lewis

Is an author, researcher, nutritionist and lecturer with a passion for helping people become healthier through nutritional awareness. He resides in southern Colorado.

docdawa@gmail.com

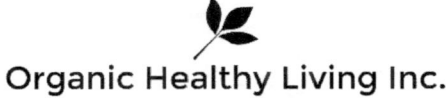

Organic Healthy Living Inc.

Publications

2015